MERIDIAN EXERCISE

FOR
SELF-HEALING

BEST
LIFE
MEDIA

Best Life Media
459 N. Gilbert Rd, Ste. C-210
Gilbert, AZ 85234
www.bestlifemedia.com
(928) 239-4002

Translated by Meryl (Meri) Harmon Halem and Youngsook Chang

ISBN-13: 978-1-935127-10-9
First paperback edition: June 2009

MERIDIAN EXERCISE

FOR
SELF-HEALING

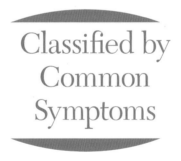

Classified by
Common
Symptoms

Back Pain * Headaches * Colds * Flu
Joint and Muscle Pain * Insomnia

ILCHI LEE

PREFACE

When you feel like you are coming down with the flu, what do you do? Do you go to the drugstore and buy an over-the-counter medication? Or do you go to the hospital? Or, knowing that there is not a cure for the flu, do you prefer to wait for the virus to run its course? Do you regret not having gotten vaccinated prior to the flu season?

Health is best maintained on a daily basis. In order to do this, one must have a clear and intimate understanding of the basic principles of how health is maintained in the body. By intimate, I do not mean an intellectual understanding. Rather, we must know our own body like we would know a loved one.

Taking care of ourselves, being in charge of our lives, is a way of saying we are worthwhile, an acknowledgment of our self-worth. We must awaken to the many inherent sensibilities and sensitivities of our body and be able to feel when we are moving toward health or away from it.

The first principle we must understand is our innate healing power. Our role as master of our body is to facilitate and enhance this process. I believe we should adopt natural self-care methods to prevent and treat common illnesses, thereby managing most daily health concerns. Our breathing, our body itself, and the life energy which flows through it become tools once we understand their principles and the basic skills for applying them.

Meridian exercise is one of the most effective self-health management skills. These exercises have a low risk of side effects and are effective, inexpensive, and easily learned and used.

Meridian exercises in this book are based on Body & Brain Yoga principles and techniques. Body & Brain Yoga provides an integrated training method that combines deep stretching exercises, meditative breathing techniques, and energy awareness practice to reach optimum health. As founder of Body & Brain Yoga, I have systemized and developed new methods for the past twenty-seven years. Body & Brain Yoga strengthens the body and its natural healing power by strengthening the fundamental life force. Meridian exercise is basic Body & Brain Yoga training as well as a comprehensive health regimen that enriches the spirit while bringing health to body and mind.

To use this book, first look through the table of contents and identify your particular symptoms. Then find the corresponding exercises to relieve your symptoms. The exercises in this book not only reduce painful symptoms, but also enhance overall health to aid in disease prevention. You may indi-vidualize your exercise program according to your particular needs.

It is most important to physically practice meridian exercises regularly. None of the methods presented here will help you unless you experience them in your body. I believe that consistent practice of meridian exercises can help maintain our health in the optimal state.

Ilchi Lee

CONTENTS

PREFACE ⋯⋯⋯⋯⋯⋯⋯⋯⋯⋯⋯⋯⋯⋯⋯ 4

CHAPTER 1.
INTRODUCTION

1. Ki, the Life Energy ⋯⋯⋯⋯⋯⋯ 10
2. What Is Meridian Exercise? ⋯⋯⋯⋯ 12
3. Benefits of Meridian Exercise ⋯⋯⋯ 14
4. Dahn-jon, Key Energy Center ⋯⋯⋯ 15
5. Abdominal Breathing ⋯⋯⋯⋯⋯⋯ 16
6. How to Use This Book ⋯⋯⋯⋯⋯⋯ 17

CHAPTER 2.
BASIC MERIDIAN EXERCISES

1. Whole Body Patting ⋯⋯⋯⋯⋯⋯ 21
2. Circulation Exercise ⋯⋯⋯⋯⋯⋯ 24
3. Abdominal Clapping ⋯⋯⋯⋯⋯⋯ 25
4. Intestine Exercise ⋯⋯⋯⋯⋯⋯⋯ 26
5. Anal Contracting Exercise ⋯⋯⋯⋯ 27

CHAPTER 3.
MERIDIAN EXERCISES FOR
SPECIFIC SYMPTOMS

1. BRAIN AND NERVOUS SYSTEM
1) Headaches ⋯⋯⋯⋯⋯⋯⋯⋯⋯ 30
2) Facial Nerve Disorders (Bell's Palsy) ⋯⋯⋯ 40
3) Autonomic Nervous System Difficulties ⋯⋯⋯ 44
4) Tingling or Numbness in the Extremities ⋯⋯⋯ 52

2. ENDOCRINE SYSTEM
1) Thyroid Disorders ⋯⋯⋯⋯⋯⋯⋯ 56
2) Diabetes ⋯⋯⋯⋯⋯⋯⋯⋯⋯⋯ 68

3. RESPIRATORY SYSTEM
1) Lung Disorders ⋯⋯⋯⋯⋯⋯⋯⋯ 78
2) Colds and Flu ⋯⋯⋯⋯⋯⋯⋯⋯ 88

4. BONE, MUSCLE, AND SKIN
1) Lower Back Pain ⋯⋯⋯⋯⋯⋯⋯ 96
2) Neck Pain ⋯⋯⋯⋯⋯⋯⋯⋯⋯ 108
3) Shoulder Pain ⋯⋯⋯⋯⋯⋯⋯⋯ 112
4) Sciatic Pain ⋯⋯⋯⋯⋯⋯⋯⋯⋯ 120
5) Arthritis ⋯⋯⋯⋯⋯⋯⋯⋯⋯⋯ 128
6) Osteoporosis ⋯⋯⋯⋯⋯⋯⋯⋯ 134
7) Skin Disorders ⋯⋯⋯⋯⋯⋯⋯⋯ 136
8) Hair Loss ⋯⋯⋯⋯⋯⋯⋯⋯⋯⋯ 146

5. HEART AND CIRCULATORY SYSTEM

1) Heart Disease ·················· 150

2) High Blood Pressure ·················· 164

3) Hypotension (Low Blood Pressure) ·········· 170

4) Stroke ·················· 174

6. DIGESTIVE SYSTEM

1) Gastrointestinal Disorders ·········· 178

2) Liver Disorders ·················· 190

3) Diarrhea ·················· 204

4) Constipation ·················· 208

5) Hemorrhoids ·················· 218

7. URINARY TRACT AND
   REPRODUCTIVE SYSTEM

1) Kidney Disorders ·················· 222

2) Bladder Infection ·················· 230

3) Stamina/Strengthening ·········· 234

8. EXERCISES FOR WOMEN

1) Exercises for Pregnancy ·········· 242

2) Postpartum Recovery ·········· 260

3) Leukorrhea ·················· 264

4) Menstrual Disorders ·········· 272

9. OTHER CONDITIONS

1) Obesity ·················· 278

2) Poor Eyesight ·················· 290

3) Impaired Hearing ·················· 294

4) Insomnia ·················· 296

5) Hangovers ·················· 304

6) Lethargy and Fatigue ·········· 310

7) Spring Fatigue ·················· 314

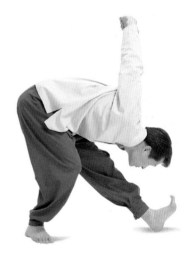

APPENDIX

1. The Spine, Main Pillar of Our Body ········ 322

2. Position of Organs and the Skeleton ······ 324

3. Meridians, Rivers of Ki Energy ·········· 326

Symptom/Benefit Index ·················· 334

chapter 1.

INTRODUCTION

1. Ki, the Life Energy

2. What Is Meridian Exercise?

3. Benefits of Meridian Exercise

4. Dahn-jon, Key Energy Center

5. Abdominal Breathing

6. How to Use this Book

1. KI, THE LIFE ENERGY

Ki, also commonly spelled *chi* or *qi*, is a fundamental concept embraced by Asian philosophy, arts, medicine, and mind-body traditions. *Ki* is the word for the vital energy that is the true essence of every creation in the cosmos. Most people begin their understanding of Ki by experiencing it as bio-energy, or the basic life force in the body.

Ki is the bridge linking the body and mind; it is the essential medium of life, moving and flowing freely. The continuous joining together and drifting apart of Ki composes the rhythm of the phenomenon of life. Everything in existence undergoes constant change. Everything around us, as well as each of our very lives, is a temporary manifestation of ki.

Although immersed in this grand flow of energy every moment of our lives, we are unable to sense its currents without properly attuned senses. Our overdependence on rational thought and language has obscured our natural ability to sense the flow of energy. However, we can regain our innate ability to feel the slight but pervasive vibrations that define our existence. It is up to us to reawaken this sense. By opening blockages in the energy pathways and reawakening our innate ability to sense energy flow, we can recover our health and natural balance. When we develop sensitivity to ki, we will be able to reach our body's potential.

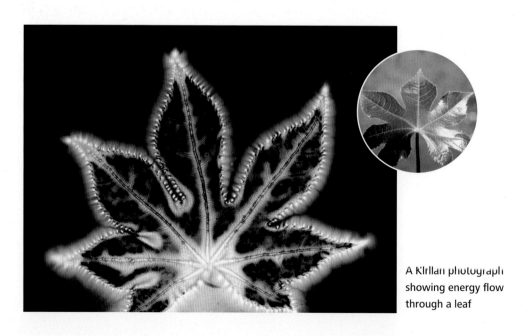

A Kirlian photograph showing energy flow through a leaf

2. WHAT IS MERIDIAN EXERCISE?

The meridian system of the body is a series of channels or pathways running from the feet to the head and from the head to the hands, transporting Ki energy. Meridians can be likened to rivers of the body. The meridian system is responsible for the distribution of Ki throughout its intricate network, nourishing and influencing body, mind, and spirit. Acupressure (or acupuncture) points, which are distributed along meridians, are portals through which energy enters and exits the body.

It is easy to understand the system of meridians and acupressure points if you imagine the body as representing land. The meridians would be the main roads while the acupressure points are the bus stops. Just as goods and merchandise are transported across a highway system, our body can supply energy to the organs and different parts of the body through meridians. If energy flows well through the meridians, it is distributed evenly throughout the body, helping the body and brain to maintain their optimal conditions.

Our body consists of twelve main meridians and eight secondary meridians. In general, only fourteen of the meridians are commonly used. Ki comes into the body through the breath. It then flows through the twelve meridians and collects in two of the eight secondary meridians—one along the back, called the Governing Vessel (Dok-maek), and one along the front, called the Conception Vessel (Im-maek). The two meet when the lips touch.

The twelve major meridians are associated with the internal organs and are named accordingly: kidneys, liver, spleen, heart, lungs, pericardium, bladder, gall bladder,

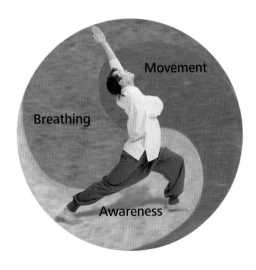

stomach, small and large intestines, and the triple burner (body temperature regulator). These twelve meridians are paired, or bilateral, and situated systematically on either side of the body. Ki flows constantly through the twelve meridians of the body, starting in the lungs and ending in the liver.

Meridian exercises are designed to open the meridian system of the body, and to balance the energy of their associated organs. The various exercises introduced in this book are derived from Body & Brain Yoga principles and methods.

Body & Brain Yoga is an integrated mind-body training method that combines deep stretching exercises, meditative breathing techniques, and energy awareness training. Its objective is to help practitioners achieve their highest level of personal potential.

The traditional name for Body & Brain Yoga is Dahnhak, which literally means "the study of energy." In Korean, Dahn refers to the primal, vital energy which is essential to all life forms, and hak refers to the study of a particular theory or philosophy. Thus, a Dahnhak practitioner is one who studies the system of energy for the purpose of overall self-development.

Meridian exercises combine proper breathing with various stretching movements. When breath is combined with body movement, metabolism can be influenced more effectively. In order to optimize the effects of meridian exercise, movement, breathing, and awareness must be harmonized. Start the movements while inhaling. Hold your breath for a moment while holding the posture and then exhale slowly while returning to the beginning position. The body should be centered at the lower Dahn-jon, or energy focus in the lower abdomen, and your consciousness should be attuned to the areas being stretched during the movements. When exhaling, imagine that the impure, stagnating energy in the body is leaving. Imagine you are having a conversation with the body and focus on the changes or sensations occurring in it.

It is important to practice meridian exercise in a way that is suitable for your body. For example, a fit person can train more intensely, whereas others should practice the movements more gently. Even ill and fragile people can benefit from gently rubbing and massaging the whole body while breathing and focusing on conscious awareness. In the beginning, try to master the movements first, rather than attempting to harmonize your breathing with them. Practice the movements according to your breathing capacity (without straining) when you are familiar enough with the movements to do them naturally.

Throughout this book, you will see various acupressure points on the body. In traditional Chinese medicine the acupressure points have poetic names. The imagery of point's name offers insight into either a point's benefits or location.

But in the West people use abbreviations that reflect the organ system influenced and the position of the meridian. See box, for the abbreviation of each meridian. Also, each point is assigned an identification number to track its placement along the body. Point location numbers, such as Ki 1, BL 8, are standard referencing system used by professional acupuncturist. See box, for key to abbreviations of the meridians. This book uses both an identification number and a Korean name to indicate each acupressure point.

ABBREVIATIONS OF EACH MERIDIAN

Bl	Bladder
CV	Conception Vessel
GB	Gall Bladder
GV	Governing Vessel
Ht	Heart
Ki	Kidney
PC	Pericardium Channel
LI	Large Intestine
Liv	Liver
Lu	Lungs
SI	Small Intestine
Sp	Spleen
St	Stomach

3. BENEFITS OF MERIDIAN EXERCISE

Physical Benefits

- Spine is lengthened and stretched
- Height can be increased by one inch.
- Practitioner develops a keen sense of awareness in distinguishing parts of the body where Ki energy has become blocked.
- Flexibility and strength are developed; stress and fatigue are lessened and released. Internal organs are stimulated, accompanied by a sense of vitality.
- Pelvis and spine are realigned, as the body reestablishes a natural symmetrical balance. Pain in these areas will diminish as symmetrical balance is optimized.
- Body's ability to break down fat cells and increase blood circulation is enhanced.
- Muscular, nervous, and circulatory systems are strengthened, and meridian system is activated.
- Toxins and stagnant energy in the body are dissipated.
- Increased sense of vitality is experienced as Ki energy is gathered in the energy center in the lower abdomen. The practitioner can experience a more vibrant voice projection. Tasks of daily living can be performed with a heightened and more robust sense of well-being.

Mental Benefits

- The body becomes very relaxed, thus calming the mind.
- Deep breathing stimulates circulation of oxygen to the brain. The head feels clear and the memory becomes sharp.
- Stress management ability is increased, as well as the ability to control emotions and thoughts. Positive attitude and joy toward life become intensified and more consistent.
- When this exercise is performed with sincerity, the practitioner can appreciate the workings of the mind/body/spirit synchronicity.
- Harmonizing of movement, breathing, and awareness is the hallmark of meridian exercise, optimizing concentration with an accompanying sense of mastery over the body. This facilitates and maximizes the self-healing process.

4. DAHN-JON, KEY ENERGY CENTER

A Dahn-jon is a place in the body where energy is gathered and stored. With enough sensitivity training, one can tangibly feel the gathering of energy in the Dahn-jon. Basically, Dahn-jon has the same definition as the word *chakra*, which means "wheel or circle" in Sanskrit.

In Body & Brain Yoga, we focus on three internal and four external Dahn-jons. The three internal Dahn-jons are located in the lower abdomen (lower Dahn-jon), in the middle of the chest (middle Dahn-jon), and in the center of the forehead (upper Dahn-jon). The four external Dahn-jons are located on each palm and on the bottom of each foot.

If a Dahn-jon is blocked, it will manifest as a physical disease or ailment. Through exercises and breath work, it is possible to facilitate the flow of energy through the Dahn-jon system of the body, resulting in overall balance and health.

When we refer to Dahn-jon in this book, it means the lower Dahn-jon, which acts as the fuel tank that stores energy for circulation throughout the body. When your lower Dahn-jon becomes strengthened, the overall energy balance of your body will be restored, amplifying your natural healing power. You will exhibit more patience and drive, developing a stronger sense of self-confidence. When you practice meridian exercises, it is always recommended to focus on the lower Dahn-jon.

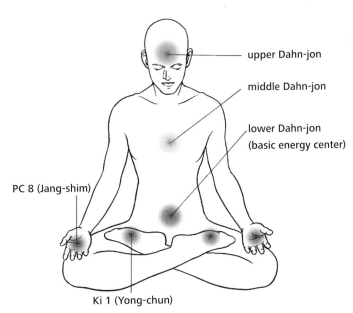

upper Dahn-jon

middle Dahn-jon

lower Dahn-jon
(basic energy center)

PC 8 (Jang-shim)

Ki 1 (Yong-chun)

Key Energy Centers in the Body

5. ABDOMINAL BREATHING

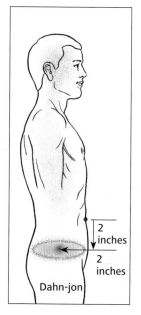

2 inches

2 inches

Dahn-jon

Deep breathing occurs naturally if we breathe with our awareness focused on our Dahn-jon. It is located roughly two inches below the navel and two inches inside the body, in the center of the abdomen.

As you do your breath work, focus your mind's attention on this area of your body. Feel your lower abdomen rising when you breathe in and falling when you breathe out. Do this slowly and concentrate on your breathing. If this method seems difficult, place one hand on your lower abdomen and the other on your chest. As you breathe, feel the hand on your lower abdomen moving while the hand on your chest stays still. This approach is called abdominal breathing or Dahn-jon breathing.

If you take time to practice this daily, soon your mind will do it automatically—abdominal breathing will simply become part of how you breathe. One part of your mind will do this deep breathing while other parts of your mind focus on other things that allow you to move through your day.

Abdominal breathing is a perfect companion to meridian exercises. After relaxing your body through meridian exercises, perform abdominal breathing for about ten to twenty minutes. It will enhance your health dramatically.

Abdominal breathing is related to the movement of the diaphragm, a dome-shaped structure that assists in breathing and acts as a natural partition between our heart and lungs on one side, and our stomach, spleen, pancreas, liver, kidneys, bladder, and small and large intestines on the other.

When we breathe deeply, our diaphragm moves downward as we inhale and upward as we exhale. The more the diaphragm moves, the more our lungs are able to expand, which means more oxygen can be taken in—and more carbon dioxide released—with each breath.

When we breathe fully and deeply, the belly, lower rib cage, and lower back expand on inhalation, thus pushing the diaphragm down deeper into the abdomen. The same structures retract on exhalation. In deep abdominal breathing, these rhythmic movements help to detoxify our inner organs, promote blood flow and peristalsis, and pump fluid more efficiently through our lymphatic system.

6. HOW TO USE THIS BOOK

Meridian exercise is different from general exercise. Meridian exercise is bringing positive energy to the body for creative energy. The synchronous movements can have far-reaching healing benefits. If you perform these exercises with honesty and sincerity, you can significantly self-heal the symptoms that cause you distress.

Look through the table of contents and identify your particular symptoms. These correspond to specific exercises you can perform to ameliorate your ailments. This book specializes not only in healing painful symptoms, but also in enhancing overall health for the body as a preventative measure. Some of the exercises for certain symptoms will be repeated in different parts of the book. You can individualize the approach according to your body condition.

If you are experiencing specific health issues, it is best to consult a trusted health care professional prior to proceeding with meridian exercises. Always listen to your body. There is no need to rush your progress or to push through your discomfort. All bodies are unique, and you will find your own level of practice naturally.

The meridian exercises will help to correct the misuse of the body from habits accrued over time. It is important to practice consistently. Some people want quick remedies and thereby become frustrated when the results are not immediate. Meridian exercises must be practiced and nurtured over time. You will feel when the condition of your body improves.

As you develop astuteness in recognizing the nuances of your body's workings and skill in deciphering a problem before it intensifies, you will continue to progress in becoming an active participant in your own self-healing.

chapter 2.
BASIC MERIDIAN EXERCISES

1. Whole Body Patting

2. Circulation Exercise

3. Abdominal Clapping

4. Intestine Exercise

5. Anal Contracting Exercise

AWAKENING THE ENERGY

When you experience tightness in the chest, you would naturally want to relieve it by patting the chest with your hands. If you sense coldness in your hands, you would automatically rub the hands together to circulate blood for accelerating warmth. The meridian exercises utilize natural body movements. When certain energy pathways or points are blocked, you pat them, open them, and get relief. The five methods described here, which could be practiced anywhere with ease, are the warm-up sequence prior to doing the meridian exercises and abdominal breathing. Twenty minutes of daily exercise will enhance your good health immensely.

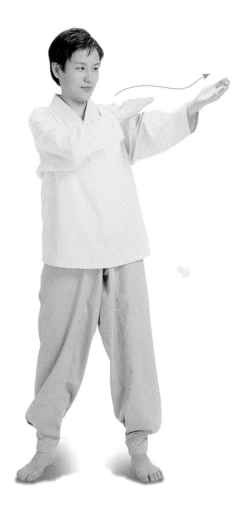

❶ Stand with your legs shoulder width apart. Begin by patting your chest with both hands. Move them back and forth across the chest, stimulating all the acupressure points on your upper chest. Increase the strength of the patting until it almost becomes a slapping movement. Extend your left arm in front of you with the palm facing up. Pat the arm with your right hand, beginning at the left shoulder, and then move down the inside of your left arm, along the wrist, palm, and fingertips. Then clap your hands ten times.

1. WHOLE BODY PATTING

Whole body patting consists of tapping the body to help circulation, open blockages, and release stagnant energy throughout the whole body. Through the patting, cells are strengthened as they are stimulated and acupressure points are opened. All age groups can perform this exercise. It is a very effective method for general health. Pat the body gently and comfortably, and allow your eyes to follow your movements.

If you feel discomfort in any area of the body you are patting, pat more lightly. This is particularly important if you experience stomach distress. Also, do not press into the area. Instead, gently rub your hands together and lightly massage that area.

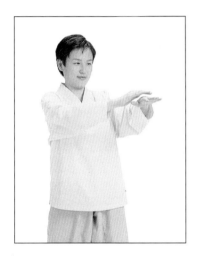

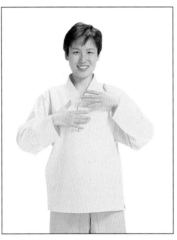

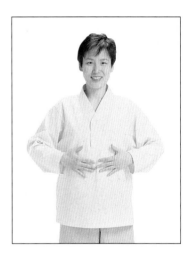

❷ Turn the left arm over so that the palm is facing down. Begin patting the back of the left hand, and then move up the back of the wrist and the outside of the arm, along the elbow, and back up to the left shoulder. Repeat for the right arm.

❸ Continue patting with both hands as you move them back to the middle of your chest.

❹ Move your hands to your solar plexus and continue patting gently.

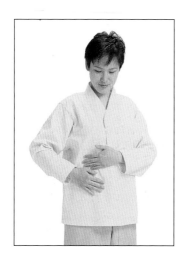
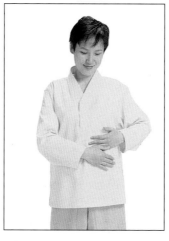

⑤ Move your hands to your stomach and liver, and continue patting.

⑥ Pat your abdomen on the left side while concentrating on the stomach.

⑦ Bend slightly from the hips as you continue patting. Move your hands so both are on the lower back over the kidneys.

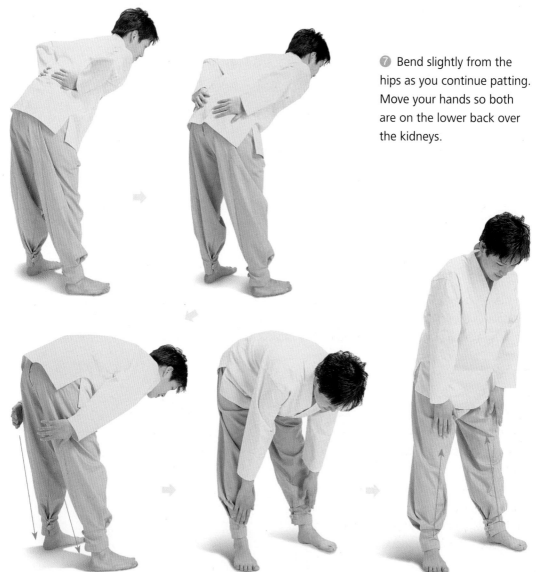

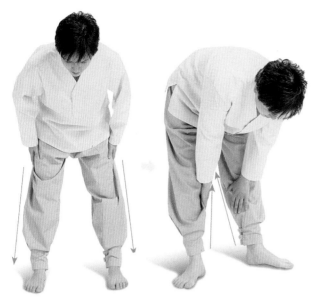

9 Bend from your hips again and tap your inner ankles. Continue to move up the inner legs toward the abdomen. Pat the abdomen 100 times in a clockwise direction.

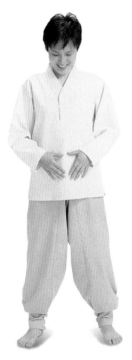

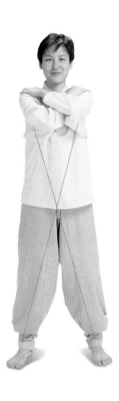

«

8 Continue to bend and pat as you move your hands down to your hips. Then pat the buttocks and continue down the backs of the legs, down to the backs of the heels, to the ankles, and around to the front and top of the feet. Continue to pat upward along the front of the legs toward the hip joints.

10 After patting your whole body, cross your arms with your hands on your shoulders. Sweep your hands down the front of your body as you uncross your arms. Sweep the rest of the body.

2. CIRCULATION EXERCISE

Circulation exercise helps to spread Ki energy throughout the body from the lower abdomen. It helps rid the body of tension and stagnant energy while strengthening cells and bones. The blood in the lower extremities circulates more freely, and this helps to slow the aging process. The vibration also allows for the distribution of oxygen to the brain, which helps brain functioning, particularly concentration and memory.

Circulation exercise is especially helpful for people who experience high blood pressure, heart disease, rheumatism, or bronchial asthma. It helps to ease the symptoms of thyroid disorders and diseases of the skin as well. If you have any of these disorders, you can increase the time spent practicing the circulation exercise up to 10 minutes per session.

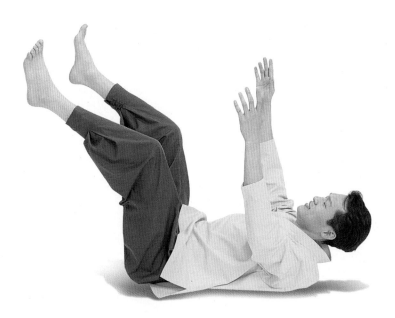

❶ Lie on the floor on your back. Extend your arms above your shoulders and your legs above your hips, bending your knees slightly. Relax the body and shake the arms and legs quickly so that the vibration reaches throughout the whole body.

❷ Do this for 1-2 minutes, and then rest. Repeat 5 times daily.

3. ABDOMINAL CLAPPING

Combined with the intestine exercise, the abdominal clapping exercise will help the intestines to become soft and flexible for abdominal breathing. This exercise not only stimulates, strengthens, and softens the intestines, but also awakens the abdomen. As you accumulate Ki energy in your abdomen, you will experience an enhanced sense of confidence and well-being.

If you eat too much meat or have poor eating habits, the food does not digest well, stagnating in the intestines. This results in constipation and other gastrointestinal upsets. Toxins can form as well, which are often responsible for the development of headaches and skin problems. Peristalsis becomes compromised and causes age acceleration. Abdominal clapping helps to lessen this condition and to restore normal peristaltic movement.

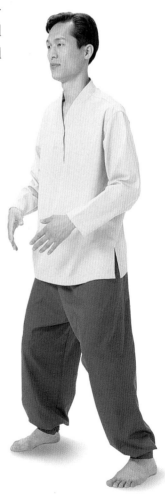

❶ Stand with your feet shoulder width apart and your knees slightly bent. Lengthen and relax your spine. Relax your shoulders, neck, and arms.

❷ Place your hands on your abdomen and begin patting the abdomen in a rhythmic motion. Increase the pressure of the patting until it becomes a striking motion, and repeat 100 times. As your abdomen becomes stronger, slowly increase the repetitions to 300. Practice daily.

4. INTESTINE EXERCISE

Proper abdominal breathing expels used Ki energy upon exhalation and acquires new Ki energy through inhalation. Abdominal breathing is only effective if the intestines are soft and flexible. Most people, when they begin meridian exercise, have stiff, hard intestines. The intestine exercise remedies this condition by increasing blood circulation to the intestines. It can remedy constipation and other digestive problems and can sometimes cause cysts in the uterus to disappear.

It is important to practice the intestine exercise on a daily basis, which is made easier by the fact that it can be performed in a variety of positions, any time and any place. You can sit, lie, or stand.

If you also tighten your rectal muscles during this exercise, you will be able to gather energy and to feel warmth much more quickly. You should not overdo this exercise in the beginning, though, because it may result in some discomfort.

Combine abdominal breathing with the intestine exercise for maximum effect. Inhale as you push your abdomen out, and exhale as you contract it. Hold each inhalation and exhalation for 2-3 seconds.

As you become more proficient, you can gradually increase the number of repetitions, up to 300.

If you experience pain in the intestines during the exercise, stop and gently rub the abdomen in a circular motion, massaging the intestines with your palms.

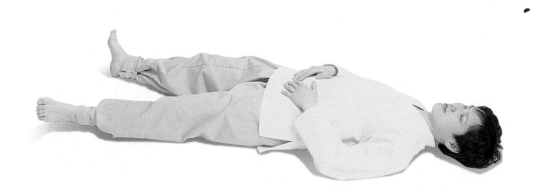

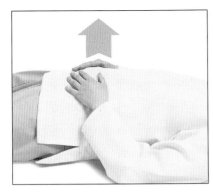

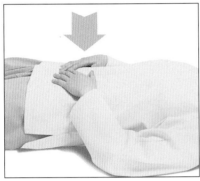

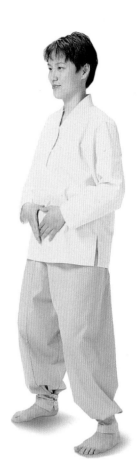

❶ Remain standing, or lie down on your back. Place your hands on your abdomen with your thumbs pointing toward the navel and your two index fingers touching together to form a triangle.

❷ Push the abdomen out until you feel pressure. Slowly and deeply pull the abdomen back in an effort to touch the spine. Repeat this movement 100 times in a rhythmic movement.

5. ANAL CONTRACTING EXERCISE

This exercise helps to stimulate the perineal area. When you sit for long periods of time, feel weak, or have a bloated stomach, the perineal/rectal area loses its elasticity, which could result in hemorrhoids, constipation, or various sexual disorders.

Anal contractions help prevent and heal hemorrhoids, vaginal itchiness, as well as bladder, urethra, uterine, prostate, reproductive, and urinary tract disorders. If acute inflammation arises, this exercise is extremely effective in relieving it. The exercise also prevents kidney disease and colon cancer as well as incontinence.

The anal contracting exercise helps to remedy impotence and erectile disorders in men, too. Furthermore, it maintains and improves elasticity in the vaginal area, thereby ameliorating female sexual disorders. Overall, this exercise can promote healthy sexual relationships.

First, inhale and hold your breath while contracting your anus all the way to the navel. Squeeze and tighten the buttocks as well. When you exhale, relax the muscles you have contracted. You could perform this without the controlled abdominal breathing, if you prefer.

chapter 3.
MERIDIAN EXERCISES FOR SPECIFIC SYMPTOMS

1. BRAIN AND NERVOUS SYSTEM

2. ENDOCRINE SYSTEM

3. RESPIRATORY SYSTEM

4. BONE, MUSCLE, AND SKIN

5. HEART AND CIRCULATORY SYSTEM

6. DIGESTIVE SYSTEM

7. URINARY TRACT AND
   REPRODUCTIVE SYSTEM

8. EXERCISES FOR WOMEN

9. OTHER CONDITIONS

HEADACHES

Headaches are often the result of greater problems disrupting the flow of energy in our body. Cool water energy and hot fire energy flow simultaneously within our body. Energy flow originates in the chest and, when the body is in balance, moves to the appropriate parts of the body to continue the balanced circulation. This natural flow of energy is called "Water Up, Fire Down." (In Body & Brain Yoga terminology, it is called Su-seung-hwa-gang.)

Water Up, Fire Down is the core principle for human health. When the human body is in balance, the cool water energy travels upward toward the head along the back side of the body (Governing Vessel/Dok-maek), while the hot fire energy flows down the front side of the body (Conception Vessel/Im-maek) to the abdomen. This constitutes a complete cycle of energy circulation. By repeating this circulation, life maintains its balance and continuity. Perhaps you have heard the expressions "I have a fire in my belly" or "Keep a cool head."

The kidneys and the heart facilitate this constant circulation with the help of the body's energy center. The kidneys generate water energy in the human body while the heart generates fire energy. When the energy flow is balanced, the Dahn-jon imparts

heat to the kidneys and sends the water energy up. This cools the brain and sends heat down from the heart.

When the water energy travels upward along the spine, the brain feels cool and refreshed. When the fire energy flows down from the chest, the lower abdomen and intestines become warm and flexible. When this energy cycles regularly, the Dahn-jon is performing its most crucial function.

If the energy flow is reversed and fire energy moves upward while water energy moves downward, then the abdomen may be cold and the neck and shoulders stiff. One may also feel "weak at heart" or fatigued. In this state, many people experience problems with digestion, including chronic constipation, tenderness in the lower abdomen, and circulatory problems.

There are two common reasons for improper action of Water Up, Fire Down. The first occurs when the Dahn-jon, which acts to draw in and store energy, is too weak to function properly. In this case, the mind becomes cluttered with incessant thought as fire energy moves upward to the brain.

Stress can also interrupt Water Up, Fire Down because it negatively affects the downward flow of energy through the chest. When this flow is blocked, energy backs up and returns to the head, causing anxiety or headaches.

When Water Up, Fire Down is in effect, your abdomen is warm while your head is cool. Your hands and feet are warm, and you have plenty of saliva in your mouth. You sense greater clarity of mind and your senses are opened. You feel positive and relaxed, and your creativity and imagination are enhanced.

The most efficient way to eliminate headaches is to recover the state of Water Up, Fire Down in your body. The following exercises are designed to balance water and fire energy and to ease your headache symptoms.

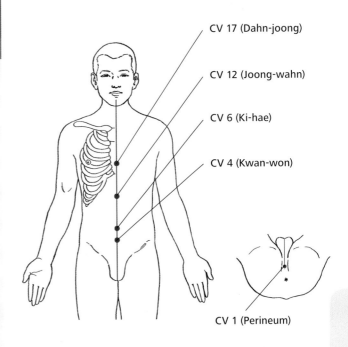

Conception Vessel (Im-maek)

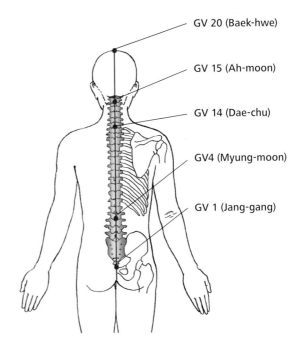

Governing Vessel (Dok-maek)

1. NECK ACUPRESSURE

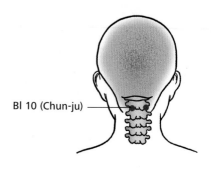

Bl 10 (Chun-ju)

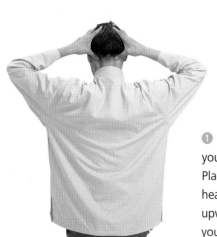

The Bl 10 acupressure points are located about one half to one inch on either side of the Ah-moon. Pressing these acupressure points helps to relieve headaches and hypertension.

❶ Kneel. Sit on your heels with your toes pointing forward. Place your hands on your head with the fingers pointing upward and the thumbs on your Bl 10 acupressure points at the base of your skull.

❷ Inhale and tilt your head to the left. Press the Bl 10 and hold for 7 seconds. Exhale. Bring your head back to center. Repeat on the right side. Perform this exercise 5 times.

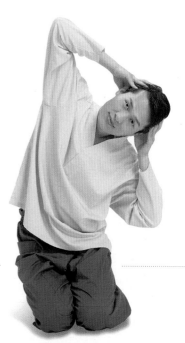

2. TOE TAPPING

❶ Lie down or sit up with your legs extended in front of you. Keeping your heels together, tap your big toes together, and then separate them so your little toes tap the floor on either side. Bring your feet up so the big toes touch again. Repeat as rapidly as you can 100 times. Increase repetitions practice.

3. STANDING ON A WOODEN PILLOW

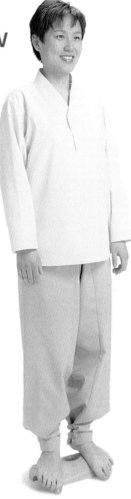

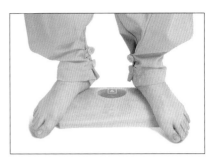

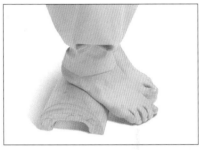

❶ Stand on the wooden pillow with bare feet. Point your toes toward the floor as much as possible. Rock your weight gently and adjust the positions of your feet to massage all parts of your feet. Continue for 5 minutes.
(Visit www.woodenpillows.com for more information about wooden pillows.)

HEADACHES

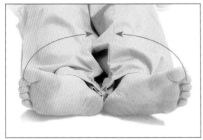

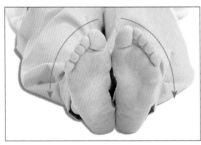

BENEFITS Helps circulation to the lower extremities and balances water and fire energy in their appropriate locations.

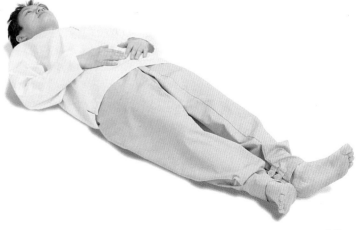

4. HEADSTAND

BENEFITS Promotes efficient blood circulation to the head and brain stem, relieving headaches. Stimulates the brain and enhances memory, concentration, and focus. Regulates hormonal functioning.

TIPS Massage the neck prior to performing a headstand. If you find balancing in the middle of the room too difficult, brace yourself against a wall.

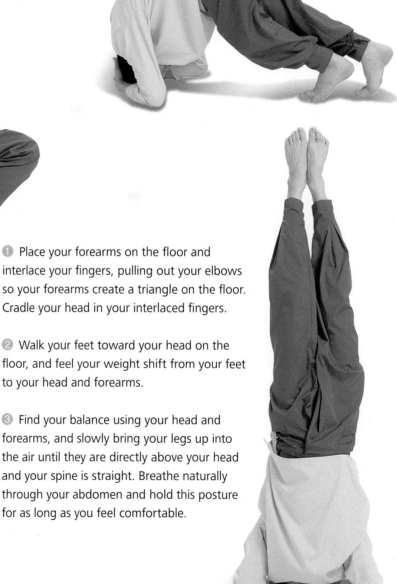

❶ Place your forearms on the floor and interlace your fingers, pulling out your elbows so your forearms create a triangle on the floor. Cradle your head in your interlaced fingers.

❷ Walk your feet toward your head on the floor, and feel your weight shift from your feet to your head and forearms.

❸ Find your balance using your head and forearms, and slowly bring your legs up into the air until they are directly above your head and your spine is straight. Breathe naturally through your abdomen and hold this posture for as long as you feel comfortable.

5. NECK MASSAGE

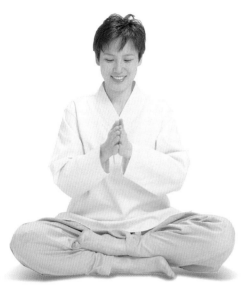

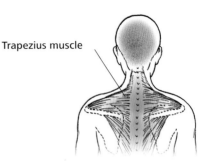

Trapezius muscle

A wide and flat muscle, shaped like a triangle, which covers the upper and back part of the neck and shoulders.

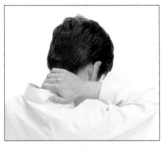

① Rub your palms together quickly to create heat. Lower your head and use your fingertips and palms to slowly squeeze and massage the back of your neck until the area has become warm and relaxed.

② Then roll your head clockwise to the right and around to the left very slowly in a circular motion. Repeat in a counterclockwise circular motion.

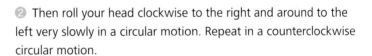

③ Cross your left arm over your chest, and place your hand on the trapezius muscle on the right side of your upper back. Massage it slowly with your fingertips. Then move your hand down your shoulder and arm, slowly massaging along the way. Repeat on the other side.

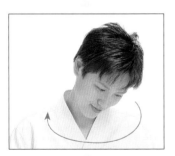

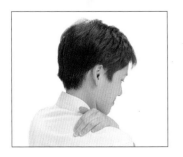

6. LEG TAPPING

BENEFITS Stimulates the Stomach Meridian and relieves stagnant energy.

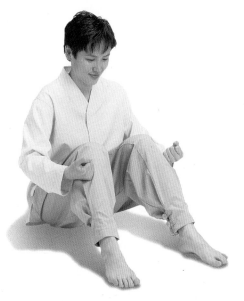

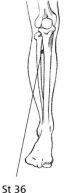

St 36
(Jok-sam-lee)

These acupressure points are located just below the knee, slightly to the outside of the shin bone, and in between the meeting point of the tibia and fibia bones. Practitioners of Eastern Medicine believe that stimulating these acupressure points enhances longevity. Patting these points aids digestion, and alleviates headaches, circulatory, and other problems in the legs, as well as respiratory, cardiovascular, and nasal conditions.

❶ Sit on the floor with your legs in front of you, feet shoulder width apart, and knees bent comfortably. Make a loose fist with each of your hands. Using the pinky side of your fists, pat the St 36 acupressure points 100 times.

7. PRESSING THE TEMPLES

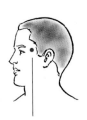

Tae-yang

Located in the temples.

TIPS Press these acupressure points with a comfortable pressure, not too firmly.

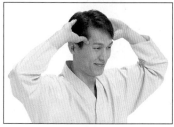

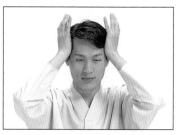

Pad of the hand.

❶ Place your hands on your head with the fingertips pointed backward and the thumbs resting on your temples. Using your thumbs, slowly squeeze the Tae-yang acupressure points in your temples with a comfortable pressure. Repeat 5 times.

❷ Rotate your hands so the fingertips point upward and the pads of the hands are resting on the temples. Using the pads of the hands, lightly tap the temples 30 times.

8. HEAD STIMULATION

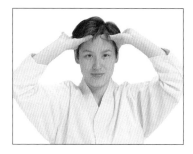 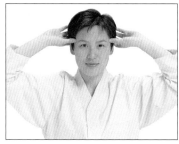 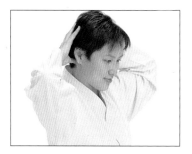

❶ Place your hands on your head with the thumbs close together at the hairline. Press your thumbs in to lightly massage your scalp at the hairline. Move your thumbs apart and continue to massage lightly along the hairline. End at the back of the neck.

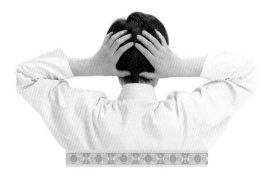 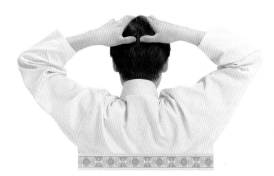

❷ Massage the back of the neck with your thumbs, starting at the hairline and moving upward to the top of the head and forward to the front hairline, where STEP 1 started. Repeat STEPs 1 and 2.

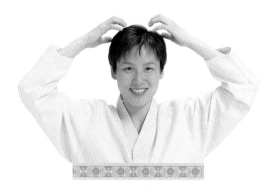

❸ Lightly tap your entire head with your fingertips, beginning at the top, moving toward the back, and then to the temples, and finally to the forehead. Feel each area as you tap and continue to breathe out through your mouth. Spend 10-20 seconds tapping each area.

9. CRANE POSTURE

BENEFITS Clears head and balances right and left hemispheres of the brain, enhancing concentration. Improves nervous system function.

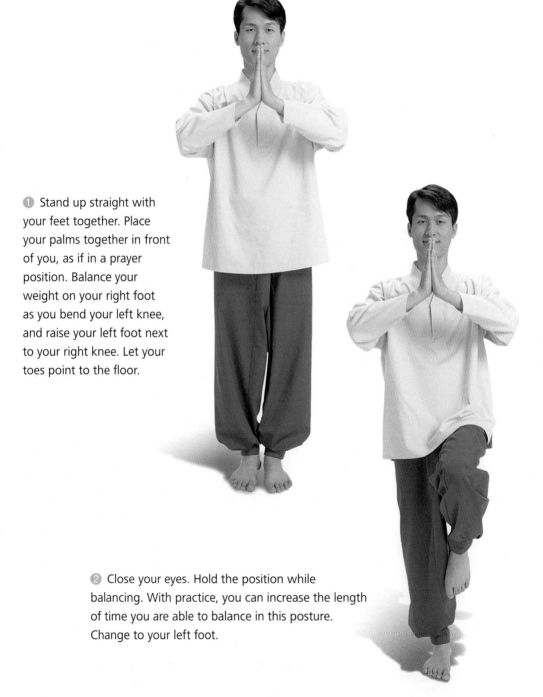

❶ Stand up straight with your feet together. Place your palms together in front of you, as if in a prayer position. Balance your weight on your right foot as you bend your left knee, and raise your left foot next to your right knee. Let your toes point to the floor.

❷ Close your eyes. Hold the position while balancing. With practice, you can increase the length of time you are able to balance in this posture. Change to your left foot.

10. SOLE PATTING

BENEFITS Significantly bolsters brain function. The feet are like a "second heart." They are vital in orchestrating proper blood circulation. When the soles of the feet are stimulated, you will begin to notice a heightened sense of clarity, focus, and concentration.

❶ Sit on the floor with your legs extended in front of you. Bend one leg and bring the ankle over the knee of the other leg.

❷ Make a fist with your thumb tucked inside your hand. With the pinky side of your fist, pound the sole of your foot strongly 30 times. Alternately, you could use a wooden stick to press the soles of the feet. Pay attention to your Ki 1 (Yong-chun) acupressure points. Repeat with the other foot.

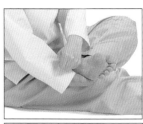
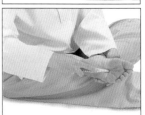

11. FINGER STRETCHING

BENEFITS Increases blood circulation to the fingers, which enhances the transport of energy throughout the body. Heightens mental clarity.

TIPS Perform this exercise quickly, exerting force with each finger stretch. When you are fatigued, perform this stretch less strenuously.

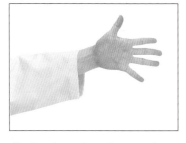

❸ Continue thrusting out the other fingers of your hand, ending with your thumb. Stretch them all out wide. Tuck your thumb back in and your other fingers individually until you close your fist, as in STEP 1. Repeat the sequence for 30 seconds with each hand.

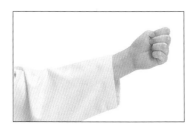

❶ Make a fist with your thumb tucked inside your hand.

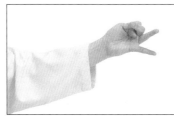

❷ Thrust out your pinky finger, tensing the muscles in your hand and forearm.

1. FACIAL TOUCH

FACIAL NERVE DISORDERS (Bell's Palsy)

Bell's palsy is a facial nerve disorder causing paralysis across one side of the face. The person experiences weakness of the whole side of the face, which often droops compared to the other side. The disorder involves swollen nerves, possibly due to a compromised immune system or a virus. The cause is unknown, although it is believed to stem from extreme fatigue or stress.

When pressure is applied to the correct acupressure points in the face, symptoms of Bell's palsy can dissipate. However, if the symptoms have persisted for more than six months, they will be more difficult to treat.

The following exercises are specifically designed to treat these symptoms and to prevent them from occurring altogether. Try to reduce exposure to the cold by covering the face, and minimize undue stress and fatigue in your daily bl.

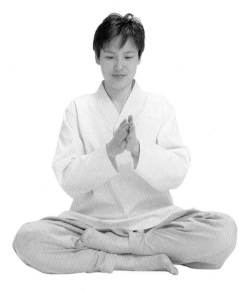

❶ Inhale from your lower abdomen. Hold your breath while you rub your palms together to create heat.

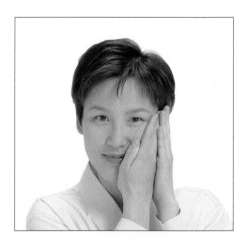

❷ Place both palms on the palsy-affected area. Exhale slowly. Repeat for 5 minutes every morning and evening

2. FACIAL STIMULATION

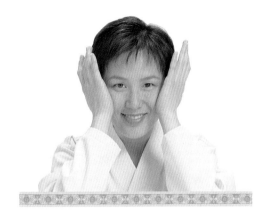

❶ Place your palms on your cheeks Press and move in a circular motion. Pay special attention to the area around the jaw.

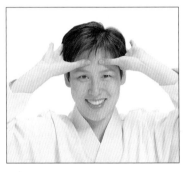
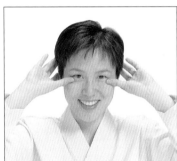

❷ Place your hands on your head with your thumbs close together in the middle of the forehead. Apply pressure with your thumbs. Remove the pressure and move your thumbs slightly farther apart. Reapply pressure. Continue moving your thumbs around the eyes, reapplying pressure at intervals.

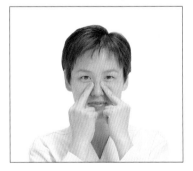
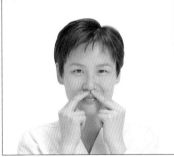

❸ With your index and middle finger of each hand, press on either side of the bridge of your nose. Move your fingertips down the sides of the nose and reapply pressure. Continue around the nose, and then around the mouth, and proceed to the chin. Spend 10 minutes performing this exercise.

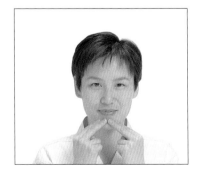

3. FACIAL REJUVENATION POSTURE

BENEFITS Helps to alleviate facial paralysis and shoulder pain while clearing and strengthening the lungs.

TIP Begin this exercise by performing for only a couple of minutes per day. Then progress up to 20 minutes per day.

FACIAL NERVE DISORDERS

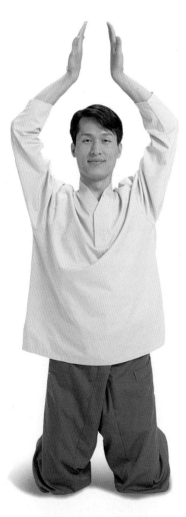

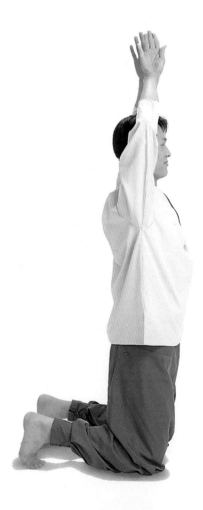

❶ Stand on your knees on the floor with your toes pointing forward. Bring both arms above your head, with the backs of your hands facing each other overhead. Open your chest.

❷ Keep your spine straight and breathe normally for up to 20 minutes.

4. FACIAL STRETCH

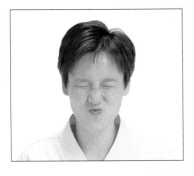 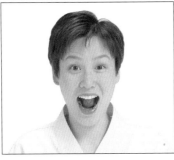 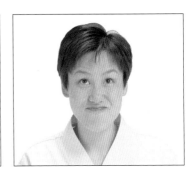

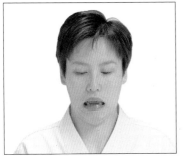 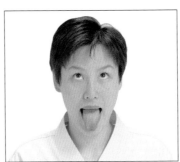

❶ Contract your facial muscles, including your eyes, nose, and mouth. Release with an open-mouthed smile, eyes wide open.

❷ Continue to move your face in various ways as shown in the pictures. Look into the mirror while practicing this exercise.

5. CHIN CIRCLES

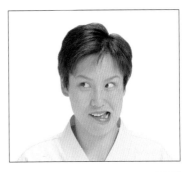

❶ Concentrate on keeping your head straight and relaxing your neck and shoulders while performing this exercise. Open your mouth and move your chin to the right, as you simultaneously shift your eyes to the left.

❷ Then move your chin to the left, simultaneously shifting your eyes to the right.

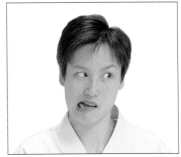

AUTONOMIC NERVOUS SYSTEM DIFFICULTIES

The autonomic nervous system governs most of our bodily functions and encompasses the sympathetic and parasympathetic networks.

The sympathetic nervous system activates the "fight or flight" response when we are in potentially harmful situations, triggering increased heart rate and blood pressure, sweating, inhibition of digestion, and release of energy stores for use by the large muscle groups. In contrast, the parasympathetic nervous system activates the "rest and digest" function, relaxing the muscles and sending blood to digestive organs to promote proper absorption of energy.

The vagus nerve is part of the parasympathetic nervous system, extending from the medulla in the brain to the base of the spine, forming a network of vital links to the heart, liver, lungs, and other organs.

Most noteworthy about this vital nerve is the correlation between its function and the phenomena people experience when they activate the Water Up, Fire Down energy principle. Warmth in the abdomen, calm heart, teary eyes, and watering mouth are believed to represent increased parasympathetic activity—a rest-and-digest workout for our autonomic nervous system.

Studies show that many natural health practices, including deep abdominal breathing and acupuncture, can stimulate activity in the parasympathetic nervous system. The meridian exercises on the following pages aim to enhance parasympathetic responses and to balance and harmonize the two autonomic nervous system branches, thus creating an optimal state of health.

1. PENDULUM SWING

BENEFITS This exercise helps to release stagnant energy from the upper body while balancing the autonomic nervous system.

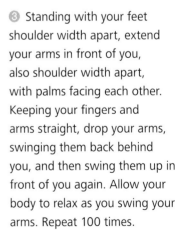

① Stand with your feet parallel and shoulder width apart. Center your weight on the soles of your feet. Extend your right arm at shoulder height to the right side, palm down. Bend the elbow of your left arm and bring your forearm across your body, palm up.

② Keep your arms, neck, and shoulders relaxed. Keeping your head centered and your gaze straight ahead, move your arms like a pendulum, dropping and swinging them up on the left side of your body, pausing at the top so your arms mirror the starting position. Continue to swing your arms 50-100 times.

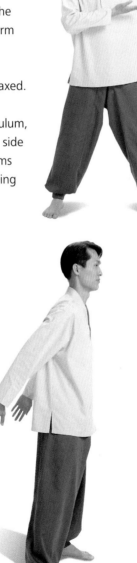

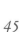

③ Standing with your feet shoulder width apart, extend your arms in front of you, also shoulder width apart, with palms facing each other. Keeping your fingers and arms straight, drop your arms, swinging them back behind you, and then swing them up in front of you again. Allow your body to relax as you swing your arms. Repeat 100 times.

2. TIGER FEET POSTURE

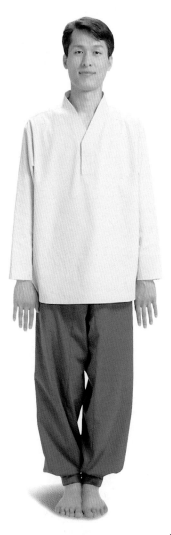

❶ Stand with your feet together and your arms at your sides, palms facing backward.

❷ Imagine holding the mouth of a jar with your fingertips, bending your wrists and spreading your curled fingers wide apart. Tense your fingertips as if to hold onto the jar.

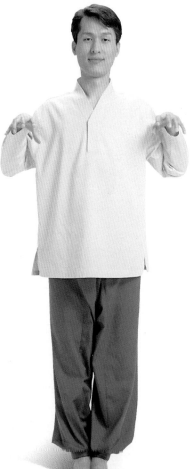

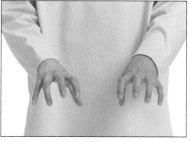

❸ Inhale. Raise your hands to chest level, hold, and release. Repeat several times.

3. MOVING A JAR

TIP Concentrate on your spine while performing this movement.

❶ Stand with your legs wide apart, knees bent and feet parallel, spine straight. Raise your arms to chest level, bending them at the elbows and allowing your index fingers and thumbs to touch, forming a triangle with your palms face down. Move your hands away from you slightly, so your arms form a circle.

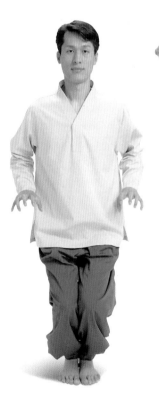

❷ Imagine you are holding a jar in between your fingers. Inhale and, concentrating on your spine, move your arms and upper torso to the left, holding the jar in front of your chest, allowing your head and eyes to follow.

❸ Pause when you've turned as far as you can.

❹ Exhale while returning to center. Repeat STEP 2 to the right. Exhale while returning to center. Concentrate on your spine, remembering to follow the movements with your eyes. Repeat twice.

❺ Bring your feet together and your arms to your sides at the level of your lower abdomen. Spread and tense your fingers as in the Tiger Feet Posture. Maintaining a straight spine, exhale as you bend your knees and ankles. Pause and return to the beginning position. Repeat 5 times.

4. UPPER BODY LIFT

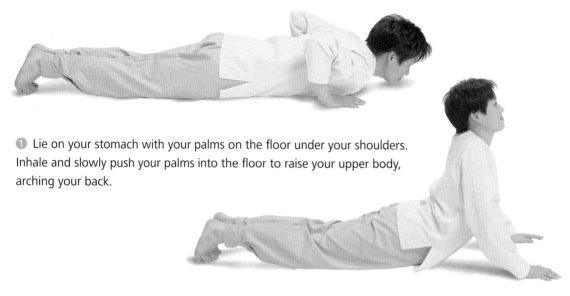

① Lie on your stomach with your palms on the floor under your shoulders. Inhale and slowly push your palms into the floor to raise your upper body, arching your back.

② As you raise your upper body, raise your head up, and hold it in this position while concentrating on your spine.
③ Exhale and return to STEP 1. Repeat 3 times.

5. HEAD STIMULATION

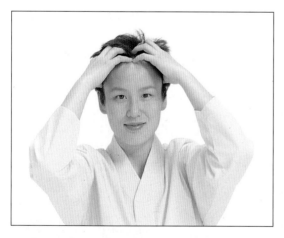

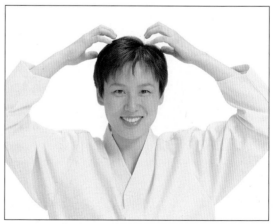

① Place your fingertips on your head with your fingers apart. Beginning at the forehead, comb your fingertips backward over your scalp. Repeat 36 times.

② Smile and tap your head with your fingertips for one minute, moving all around your scalp.

6. CHEST OPENING BACK BEND

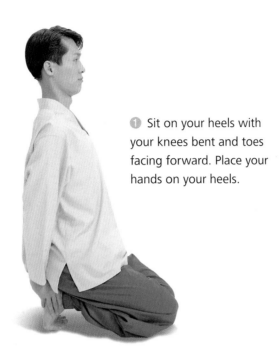

❶ Sit on your heels with your knees bent and toes facing forward. Place your hands on your heels.

❷ Lift your buttocks, open your chest, and tilt your upper torso backward. Then tilt your head backward. Experience your chest opening.

❸ Return to STEP 1 gently and slowly. Repeat the movement 3 times.

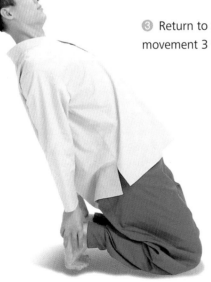

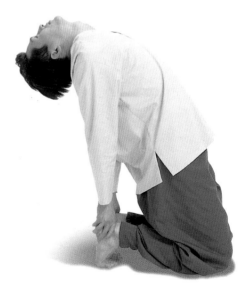

7. SITTING FORWARD BEND

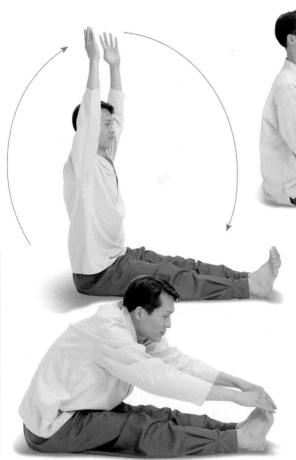

1 Sit with your legs together, extended straight out in front of you. Concentrate on straightening your spine. Place your hands on your knees.

2 Bring your arms backward in a circular motion, first toward your hips, first behind you, and then circling up over your head. Following the momentum of your arms, bend your torso and reach your fingertips toward your toes. Repeat the motion 10 times.

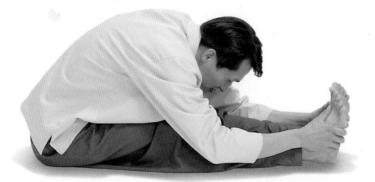

3 On the tenth repetition, hold the pose with your hands on your feet. Inhale. Concentrate on keeping your legs straight while you bend at the elbow, bringing your chest and head toward your knees. Hold this position and exhale as you try to bend more. Then breathe normally. Relax and then repeat the bend 3 more times.

8. STRADDLE WITH FORWARD BEND AND HIP LIFT

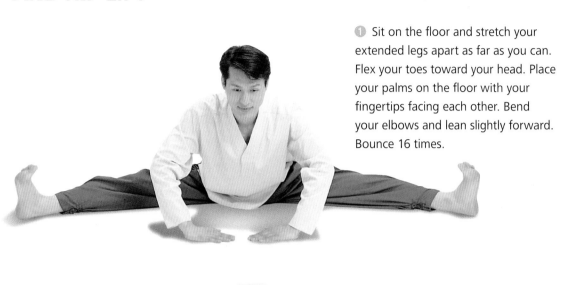

❶ Sit on the floor and stretch your extended legs apart as far as you can. Flex your toes toward your head. Place your palms on the floor with your fingertips facing each other. Bend your elbows and lean slightly forward. Bounce 16 times.

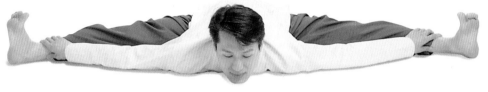

❷ With your spine straight, move your hands toward your ankles and bend more from your hips, trying to touch your chest and chin to the floor. Return to the sitting position. Repeat twice.

❸ Sit up and tilt slightly backward, palms on the floor and fingers pointing behind you. Inhale while pointing your toes. Place pressure on your heels and hands to lift your lower body. Concentrate on flexing your lower abdomen. Tilt your head backward. Exhale slowly, and gently lower your body. Repeat 3 times.

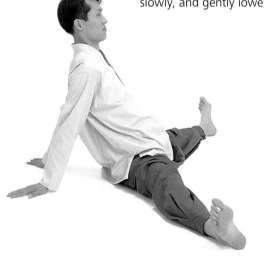

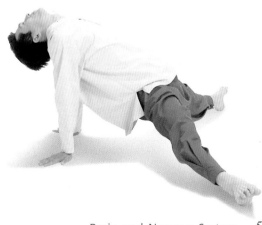

TINGLING OR NUMBNESS IN THE EXTREMITIES

The symptoms of tingling, numbness, or pain in the hands or feet arise from blockages of the somatic nervous system, which primarily governs voluntary muscle movement. Sometimes the tingling, numbness, and pain begin in the central nervous system, as when a disease is present in the brain or the spinal bone marrow. Usually, however, manifestation of these symptoms is related to peripheral nervous system blockages.

Because nerves and their actions are controlled by specific areas of the brain, the health of the brain affects the health of our nerves and muscles. When a person experiences a cardiovascular accident (CVA or stroke) in one side of the brain, the feet and hands of the opposite side of the body are adversely affected.

If you practice the following exercises, you can use Ki energy to enhance blood circulation, thereby nourishing your muscles and extremities. In addition, you can release stagnant or toxic energy that has accumulated in the peripheral nervous system areas. Tingling, numbness, or pain in your hands and feet will be alleviated.

WHOLE BODY PATTING (P. 20)

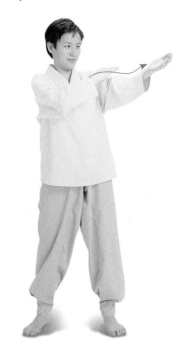

CIRCULATION EXERCISE (P. 24)

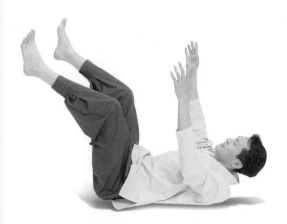

1. ARM SWINGS

TIPS Relax your body while bouncing. Repeat as you please. This exercise is most beneficial when performed as a graceful, slow dance.

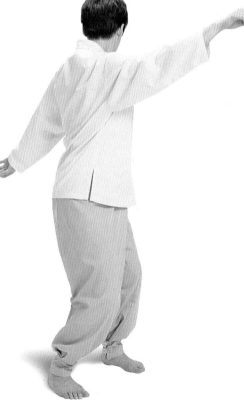

❶ Stand with your feet parallel and shoulder width apart, knees slightly bent. Extend one arm in front of you, slightly above shoulder level. Extend the other arm behind you at a comfortable height.

❷ Swing your front arm down and behind you at the same time as you swing your back arm up and in front of you. Simultaneously, turn your head to follow the movement of the hand moving behind you with your eyes.

❸ Continue this swinging movement while bouncing your knees gracefully.

2. SUPERMAN POSTURE

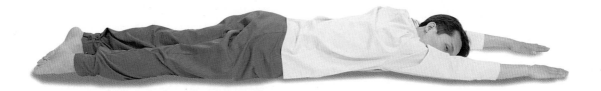

❶ Lie on your stomach with your arms reaching out in front of you.

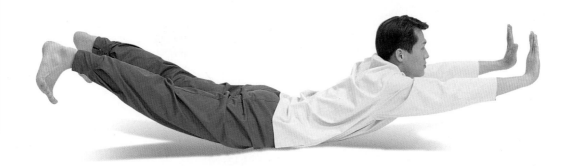

❷ Inhale. Lift your head up. Looking straight ahead, arch your back and lift your hands and feet. Tense your wrists and ankles so they make 90-degree angles with your arms and legs. With advanced practice, you can employ abdominal breathing to enhance the benefits of this exercise.

❸ Exhale. Relax your body as you let it return to the floor. Repeat.

3. BOAT POSTURE

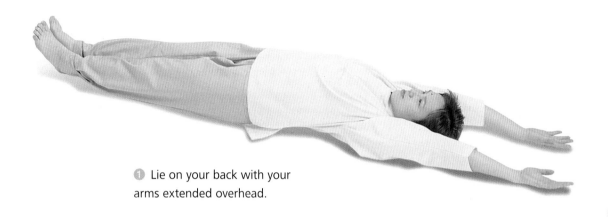

❶ Lie on your back with your arms extended overhead.

❷ Lift your head and arms to about a 45-degree angle to your torso at the same time as lifting your legs to the same angle, so that your body resembles a boat. Hold for 30 seconds and then rest for 30 seconds. Repeat for 10 minutes or more.

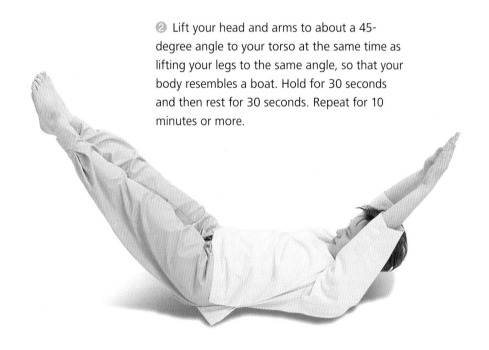

THYROID DISORDERS

The thyroid is a small, butterfly-shaped gland inside the neck and in front of the breathing airway. Thyroid hormones regulate metabolism, helping the body break down food into energy, using that energy immediately or storing it for the future.

Thyroid hormones influence virtually every organ system in the body. They tell organs how quickly or slowly they should work. Thyroid hormones also regulate the consumption of oxygen and the production of body heat.

Too much thyroid hormone from an overactive gland, called hyperthyroidism, speeds up the body's metabolism. Too little thyroid hormone from an underactive gland is called hypothyroidism. In hypothyroidism, the body's metabolism is slowed.

The following exercises will help to restore balance in thyroid functioning.

1. EXPANDING THE CHEST AND PUSHING THE ARMS

TIPS When you push your arms out, hold the wrists at a 90-degree angle. Turn your head and follow the arm behind you with your eyes. When you turn your head, you should feel tension as your neck stretches.

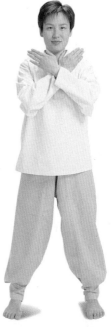

❶ Place your feet parallel and shoulder width apart. Cross your arms in front of your chest, with your palms facing your chest but not touching it.

CIRCULATION EXERCISE (P. 24)

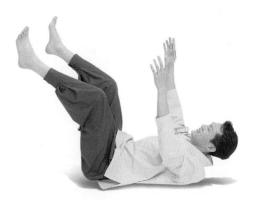

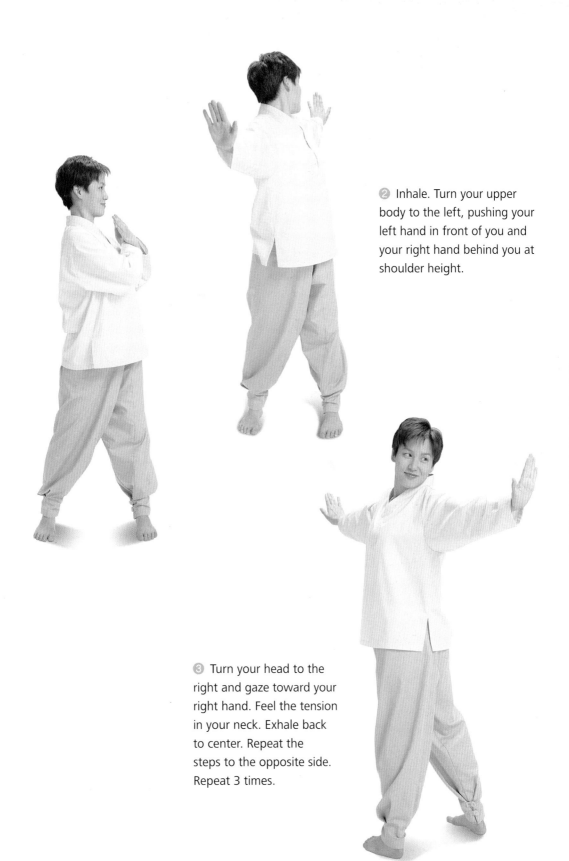

❷ Inhale. Turn your upper body to the left, pushing your left hand in front of you and your right hand behind you at shoulder height.

❸ Turn your head to the right and gaze toward your right hand. Feel the tension in your neck. Exhale back to center. Repeat the steps to the opposite side. Repeat 3 times.

2. STANDING FORWARD BEND

BENEFITS Stimulates the Urinary Bladder Meridian and balances thyroid functioning. Energizes the Conception Vessel (Dok-maek), enhancing blood circulation to the heart. Optimizes functioning of the arm and shoulder muscles, liver, and other organs.

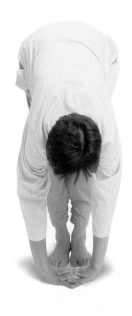
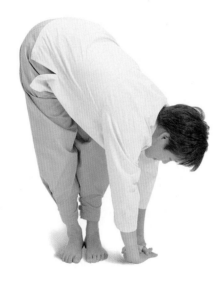
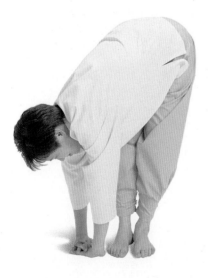
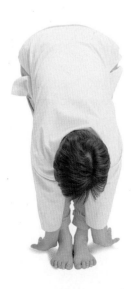

❶ Stand with your feet together. Extend your arms in front of you, and interlace your fingers. Inhale as you bend your upper body from your hips and reach your interlaced fingers toward the floor. Bounce gently. Keep your knees straight, but not tensed. Try to touch your palms to the floor in front of you. Then place your palms alternately to each side of your feet.

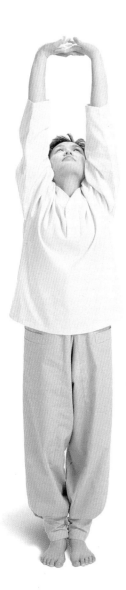

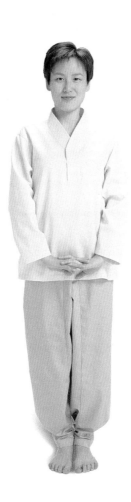

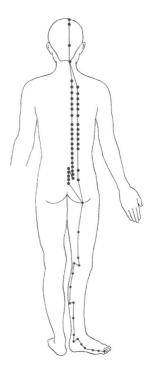

Bladder Meridian

❷ Raise your upper body to standing position with your fingers still locked. Stretch your arms above your head, palms facing the sky, and tilt your head back. Follow the stretch with your eyes and look up at your hands. Exhale and bring your hands down to your lower abdomen.

3. STRETCHING TOWARD HEAVEN

❶ Stand with your feet shoulder width apart. Make fists with your hands and bend your arms as if to flex your biceps.

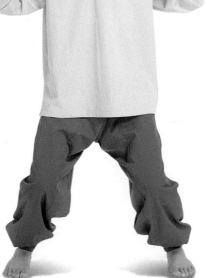

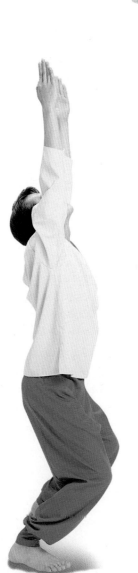

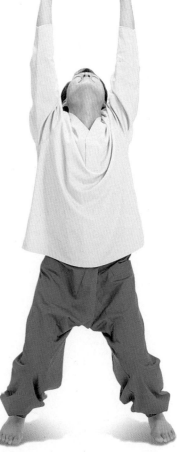

❷ Inhale, bend your knees, and stretch both arms above your head. Tilt your head back and extend your fingers upward.

❸ Keep your spine straight as you stretch your fingers up toward the sky. Follow with your eyes. Exhale. Return to STEP 1. Repeat twice.

4. HEAD LIFT

BENEFITS This exercise helps to channel Ki energy through your neck to your brain, stimulating the thyroid gland for higher production of the thyroid hormone.

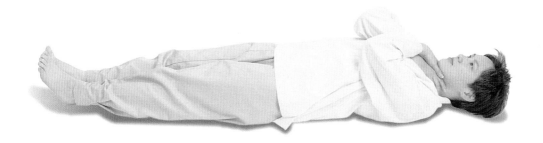

❶ Lie on your back. Open both hands and place one, and then the other, on the front of your neck.

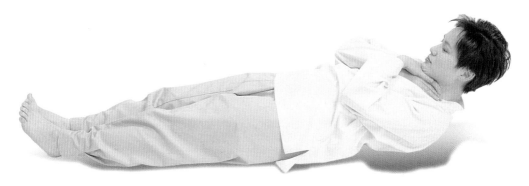

❷ Inhale. Lift your head as you push your chin toward your chest. Hold this position for 10 seconds while you gently squeeze your neck with your hands.

❸ Exhale through your mouth and return to STEP 1. Repeat one more time.

5. LIFTING LEGS OVERHEAD

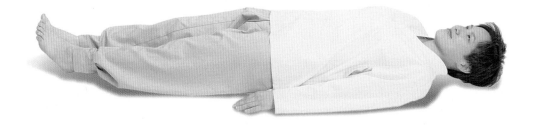

❶ Lie on your back. Breathe normally.

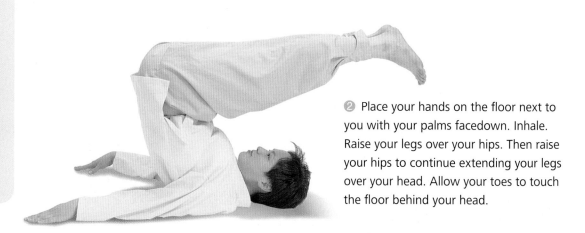

❷ Place your hands on the floor next to you with your palms facedown. Inhale. Raise your legs over your hips. Then raise your hips to continue extending your legs over your head. Allow your toes to touch the floor behind your head.

❸ Hold this position for a few seconds. Exhale. Return to STEP 1. Repeat 3 times.

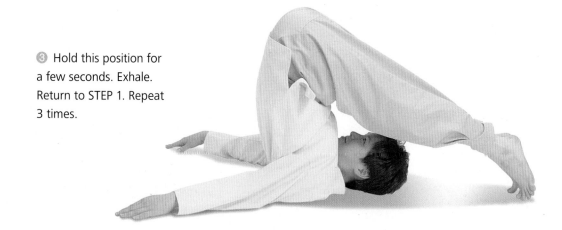

6. BACKWARD TILT

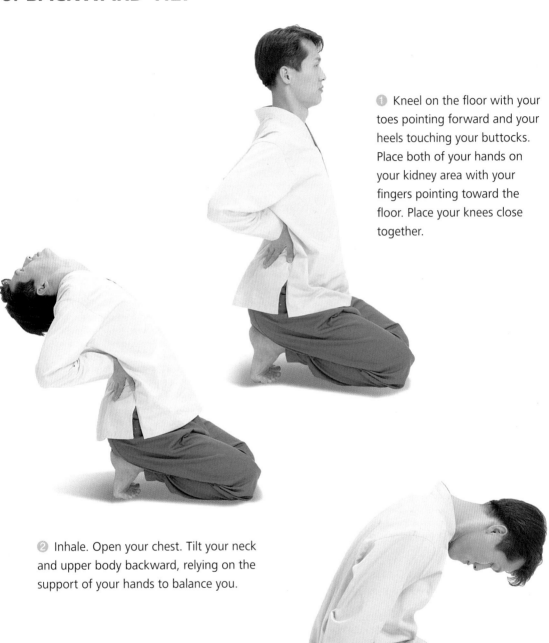

❶ Kneel on the floor with your toes pointing forward and your heels touching your buttocks. Place both of your hands on your kidney area with your fingers pointing toward the floor. Place your knees close together.

❷ Inhale. Open your chest. Tilt your neck and upper body backward, relying on the support of your hands to balance you.

❸ Exhale. Bend your upper body forward and relax your neck, so your chin falls toward your chest. Place your hands on the soles of your feet. Repeat again.

7. LUNGE WITH HEAD LIFT

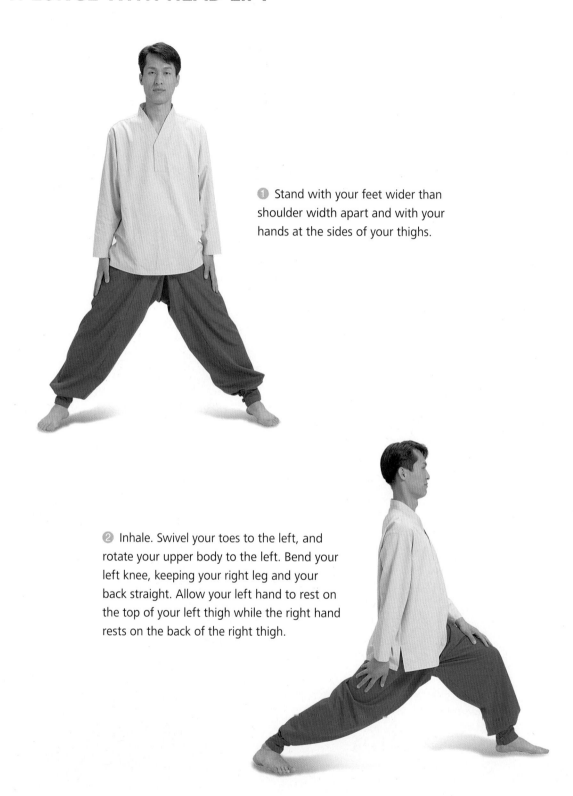

❶ Stand with your feet wider than shoulder width apart and with your hands at the sides of your thighs.

❷ Inhale. Swivel your toes to the left, and rotate your upper body to the left. Bend your left knee, keeping your right leg and your back straight. Allow your left hand to rest on the top of your left thigh while the right hand rests on the back of the right thigh.

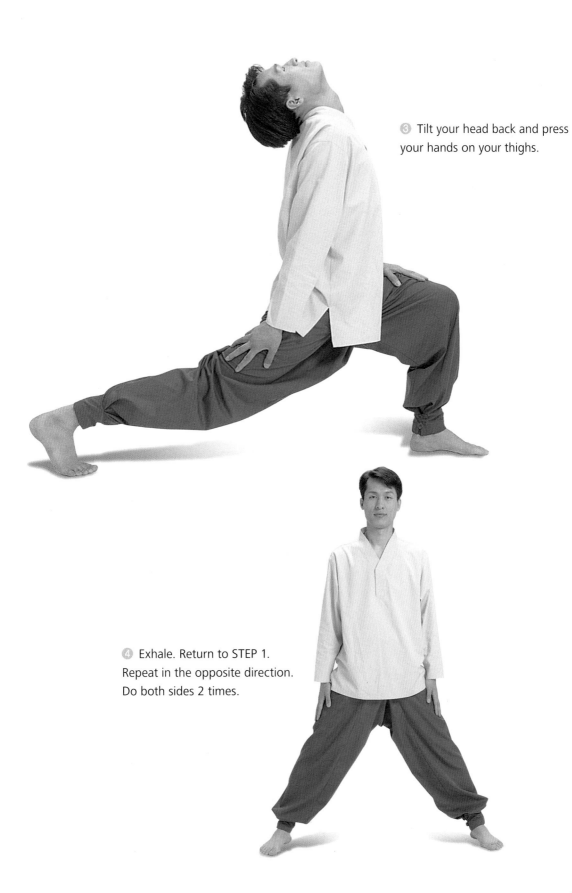

③ Tilt your head back and press your hands on your thighs.

④ Exhale. Return to STEP 1. Repeat in the opposite direction. Do both sides 2 times.

8. ARM TWIST

TIP You can perform this exercise standing or kneeling.

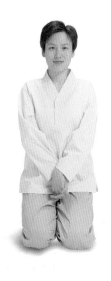 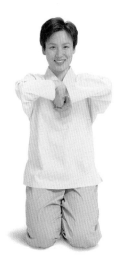 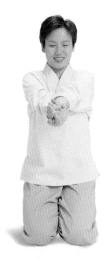

① Cross your wrists, and interlace your fingers.

② Inhale. Bend your elbows and bring your hands up and toward your chest. Continuing the movement, extend your arms out in front of your chest. Lower your hands to your lower abdomen.

③ Open your chest and tilt your head backward, keeping your back straight.

④ Exhale. Return to STEP 1. Switch the positions of your hands and repeat. Do this exercise twice in each hand position.

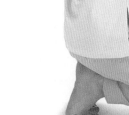

9. BACKWARD NECK TILT

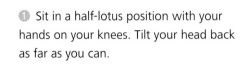

❶ Sit in a half-lotus position with your hands on your knees. Tilt your head back as far as you can.

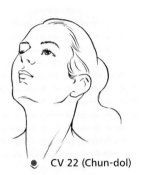

CV 22 (Chun-dol)

Acupressure point located in the divot at the bottom of the neck in the front, just below the voice box.

❷ Open your mouth. Concentrate on the CV 22 acupressure point in your neck. Keeping your head tilted back, relax your jaw so it naturally drops down like a gentle yawn. Then allow your teeth to gently touch each other. Repeat 36 times.

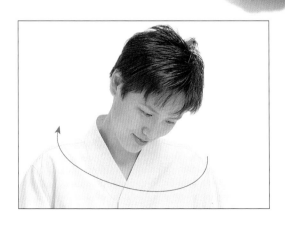

❸ Let your head drop to the right side, stretching the left side of your neck. Rotate your head very slowly in a circular motion, clockwise and then counterclockwise , to relax your neck muscles.

DIABETES

Diabetes is a disorder of the metabolism—the way our bodies use digested food for growth and energy. Most of the food we eat is broken down into glucose in the digestion process, which then passes into the bloodstream. There, insulin helps cells to absorb the glucose and transform it into energy.

When we eat, the pancreas automatically produces the right amount of insulin to move glucose from the blood into our cells. In people with diabetes, however, the pancreas produces little or no insulin. Glucose builds up in the blood and overflows into the urine. Thus, the body loses its main source of energy even though the blood contains large amounts of glucose. Other symptoms diabetics face are high blood pressure, stress, and tension.

Meridian exercises in this book are based on the self-management principle. Abdominal breathing boosts the immune system and allows the blood to circulate, enabling the pancreas to stabilize insulin production. These exercises are likely to result in a sense of serenity in mind and body. This is enormously helpful for easing the tension many diabetics experience.

TOE TAPPING (P. 32)

BENEFIT Helps to bring fire energy down to the lower abdomen.

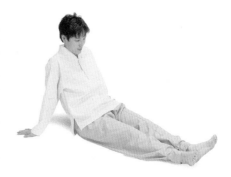

LEG TAPPING (P. 36)

BENEFITS Stimulates the Stomach Meridian and relieves stagnant energy.

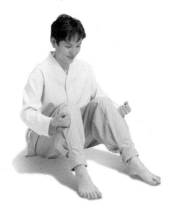

UPPER BODY LIFT (P. 48)

BENEFITS Stimulates insulin secretion and aligns spinal cord while strengthening the kidneys, bladder, and reproductive system.

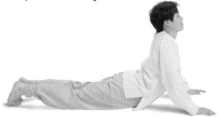

1. RAISING HANDS

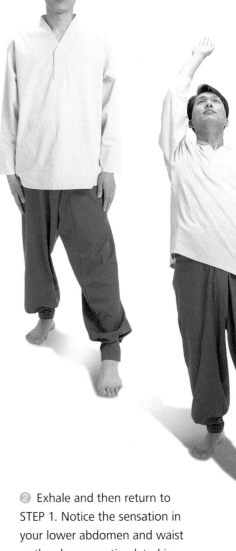

① Stand with your left foot forward. Inhale. Let your left hand rest on your left thigh, and raise your right hand toward the ceiling as you tilt your body backward, arching your back slightly and shifting your weight onto your right foot. Follow the movement of your hand with your eyes. Tilt backward as far as you can.

② Exhale and then return to STEP 1. Notice the sensation in your lower abdomen and waist as they become stimulated in this exercise.

③ Repeat twice for each side of the body.

2. SPIRAL DANCE

BENEFITS Enables joint flexibility and mobility. Strengthens autonomic nervous system while enhancing optimal organ function, supporting the immune system, and helping to prevent and treat age-related problems.

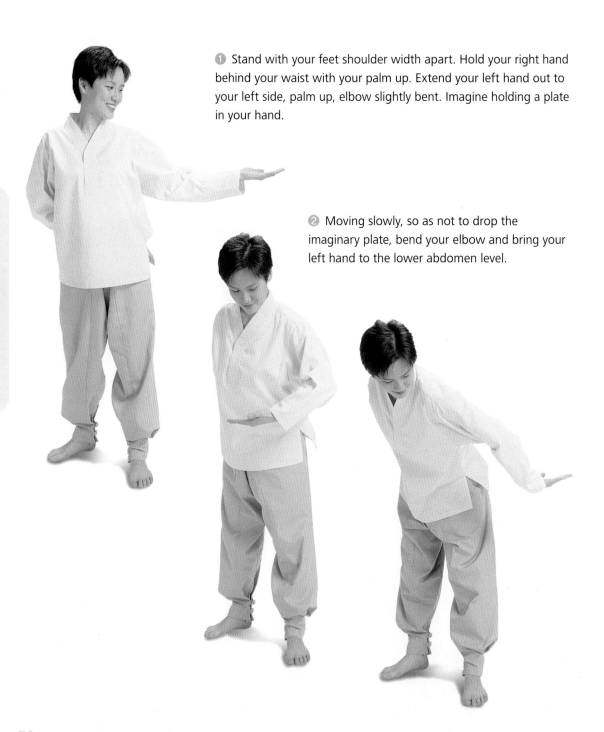

❶ Stand with your feet shoulder width apart. Hold your right hand behind your waist with your palm up. Extend your left hand out to your left side, palm up, elbow slightly bent. Imagine holding a plate in your hand.

❷ Moving slowly, so as not to drop the imaginary plate, bend your elbow and bring your left hand to the lower abdomen level.

3 Point your elbow out, and bring the plate under your arm and behind you. Then extend your arm and swing it in front of you as you bring the plate up to make a clockwise circle around your head, creating a large *S* shape that ends in a loop. Throughout the exercise, concentrate on keeping your plate balanced on your palm, and follow your hand movements with your eyes.

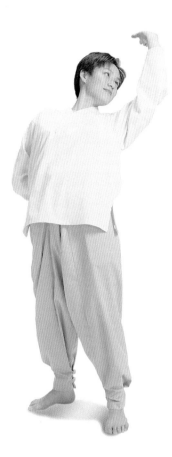

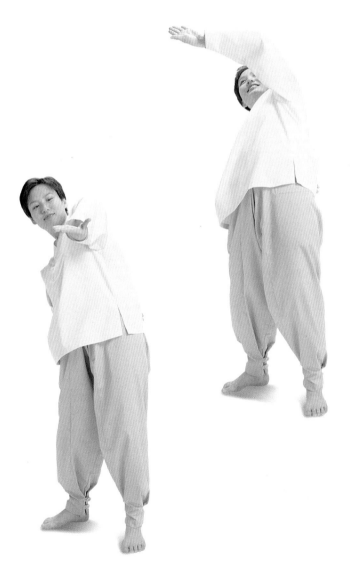

4 Alternate your hands while repeating this exercise 10 times. Progress to drawing larger circles and S shapes with practice.

3. UPPER BODY BEND AND TWIST

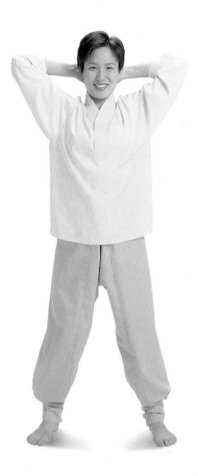

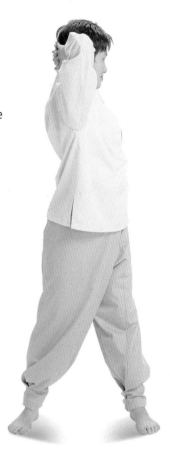

❶ Stand with feet shoulder width apart. Interlace your fingers behind your neck. Inhale while turning your upper body to the left.

❷ Bend at the waist and bring your head toward your left knee. Hold for a few seconds. Notice the stretching in your inner thighs, chest, abdomen, and waist.

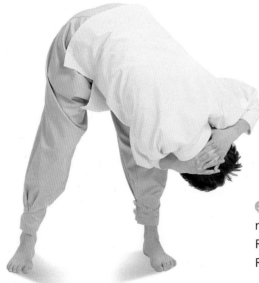

❸ Move your head and trunk toward your right knee. Exhale. Hold for a few seconds. Return to standing position, as in STEP 1. Repeat twice for each side of the body.

4. PUSH AND PULL TOE GRAB

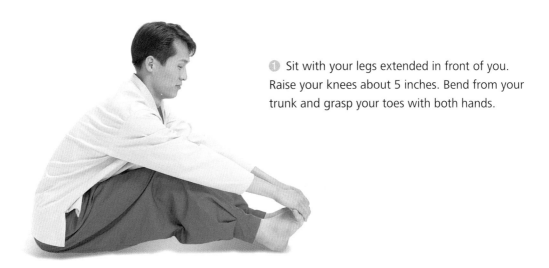

1. Sit with your legs extended in front of you. Raise your knees about 5 inches. Bend from your trunk and grasp your toes with both hands.

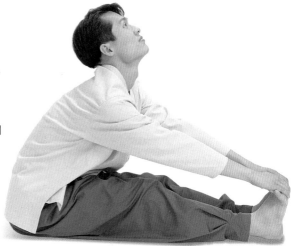

2. Inhale. Straighten your legs. Push your feet out while grasping your toes and pulling them toward you. Tilt your head back and expand your chest until you feel the stretch in your shoulder area.

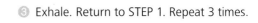

3. Exhale. Return to STEP 1. Repeat 3 times.

5. FLAGPOLE POSTURE

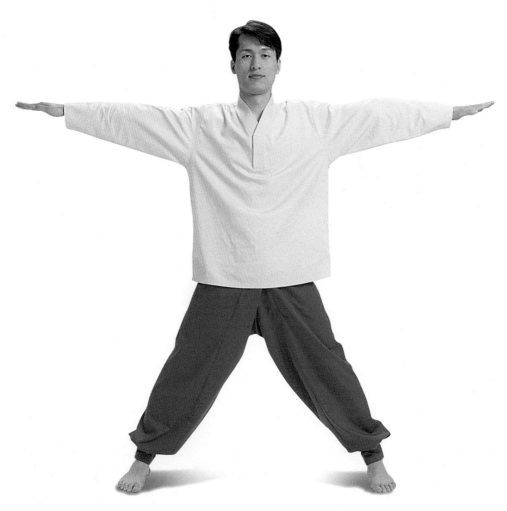

❶ Stand with feet wide apart and arms extended to the sides, palms down. Inhale. Turn your torso to the left.

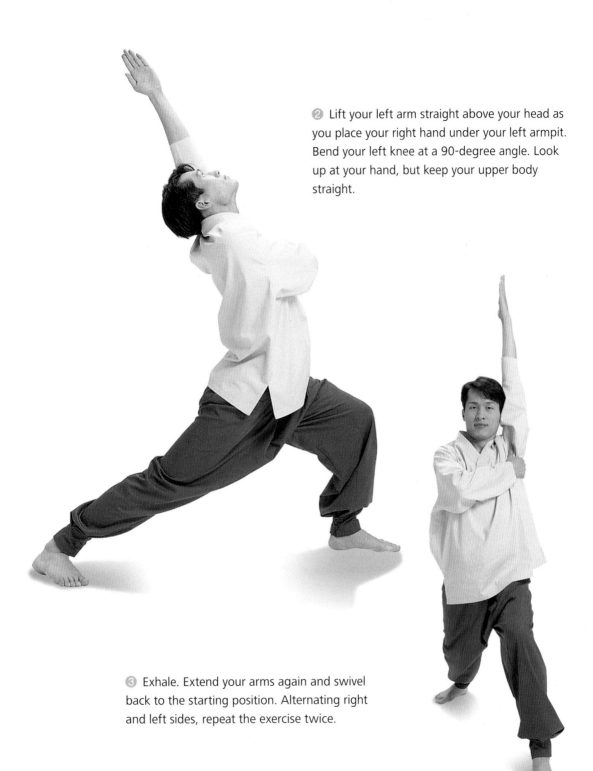

② Lift your left arm straight above your head as you place your right hand under your left armpit. Bend your left knee at a 90-degree angle. Look up at your hand, but keep your upper body straight.

③ Exhale. Extend your arms again and swivel back to the starting position. Alternating right and left sides, repeat the exercise twice.

6. SPLEEN ENERGIZER

BENEFITS Strengthens the lower abdomen and lower extremities while stimulating the Spleen Meridian. As you progress with this exercise, you will be able to more readily detect the flow of energy through the Spleen Meridian, beginning at the feet and moving up to the spleen.

TIP Keep the muscles above the navel, where your spleen and pancreas are located, relaxed.

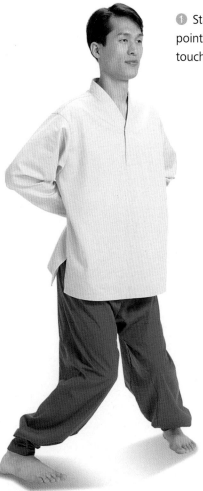

① Stand with your legs shoulder width apart, with your toes pointing inward at a 45-degree angle so your knees are almost touching. Keep your spine straight.

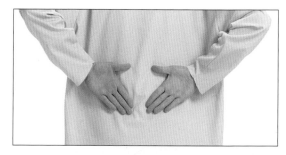

② Place both hands behind you in the kidney area, with your palms turned outward. Continue breathing out through the mouth and paying attention to the increase of circulation and warmth in the kidneys.

③ In this posture, you can notice your lower abdomen area become taut. Hold this posture for 5 minutes in the beginning. As you progress in practice, perform for 30-40 minutes.

7. CROSSING LEGS AND TWISTING

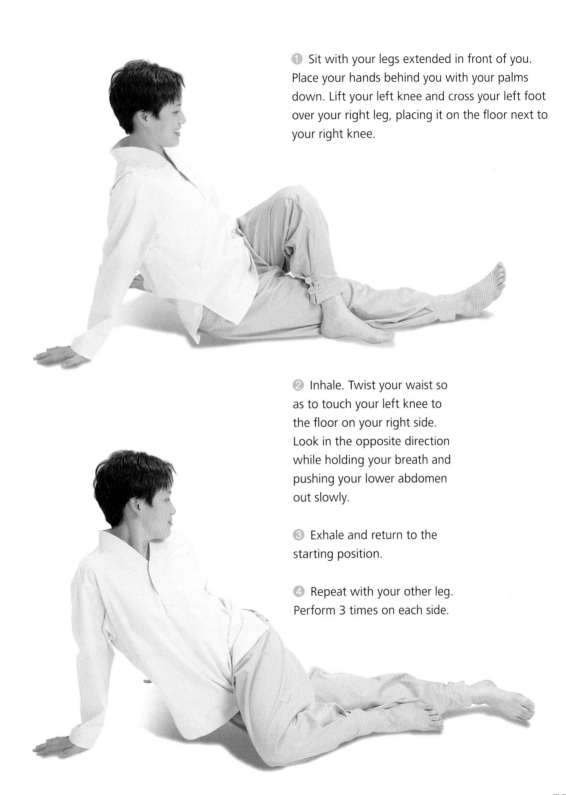

❶ Sit with your legs extended in front of you. Place your hands behind you with your palms down. Lift your left knee and cross your left foot over your right leg, placing it on the floor next to your right knee.

❷ Inhale. Twist your waist so as to touch your left knee to the floor on your right side. Look in the opposite direction while holding your breath and pushing your lower abdomen out slowly.

❸ Exhale and return to the starting position.

❹ Repeat with your other leg. Perform 3 times on each side.

LUNG DISORDERS

The primary purpose of the respiratory system is to provide oxygen to the body while ridding the system of carbon dioxide and toxic inhalants. This is accomplished through a complex series of communications and actions among the respiratory center of the brain, the chest wall, the musculoskeletal system, the nervous system, and, of course, the lungs.

The Lung Meridian is related to intense emotions. If, for example, you are very sad, the lungs can become impaired. Conditions of sadness can cause diminished lung capacity, which can lead to disorders.

Through abdominal breathing, pressure is decreased in the lungs, enabling the chest to expand, the rib cage to lift properly, and symmetry and spinal alignment to be achieved. Proficient breathing is thereby established, efficiently circulating oxygen and releasing carbon dioxide and other toxins from the body.

As you perform the exercises in this section, you will notice an overall heightened sense of well-being as your respiratory system becomes more resilient. The oxygen increase in your body will result in increased energy and concentration, enabling harmony of body, mind, and spirit.

STRETCHING TOWARD HEAVEN (P. 60)

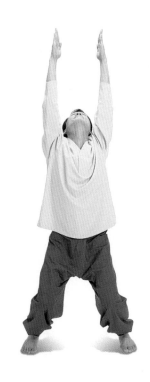

MOVING A JAR (P. 47)

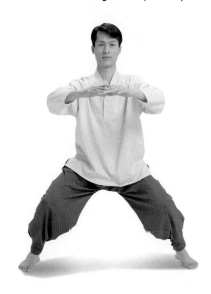

1. CLASPED HANDS FORWARD BEND

BENEFITS Expands chest to enhance and strengthen blood circulation in the lungs and endocrine system. Speeds the process through which your body releases toxins.

TIP If the lotus position is too difficult, then perform this exercise in a half-lotus position or with your legs crossed.

LUNG DISORDERS

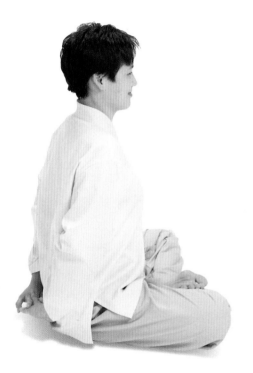
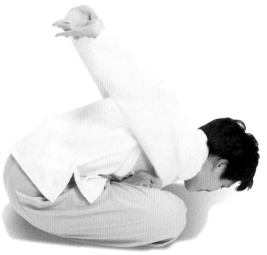

❶ Sit in a lotus position. With your arms down at your sides, join your hands behind you and interlace your fingers, palms facing down.

❷ While keeping spine lengthened, but not rigid, bend your upper body from the hips. Simultaneously lift both arms behind your back, palms facing upward.

❸ Return to STEP 1. Repeat 3 times.

2. CLASPED HANDS STRETCH AND BEND

BENEFITS Allows the spine, rib cage, and organs to achieve proper alignment to enhance the function of the respiratory system. As you stretch up toward the sky, stagnant energy is released from the shoulders and under the arms, relieving stomach distress. As you stretch toward the floor, flexibility of your neck, spine, and waist is improved.

TIPS When you push with both arms above your head toward the sky, follow the movement with your eyes. However, if dizziness occurs, or you have a history of anemia or hypertension, then fix your eyes straight ahead. Do not force this stretch. Rather, proceed gently.

LUNG DISORDERS

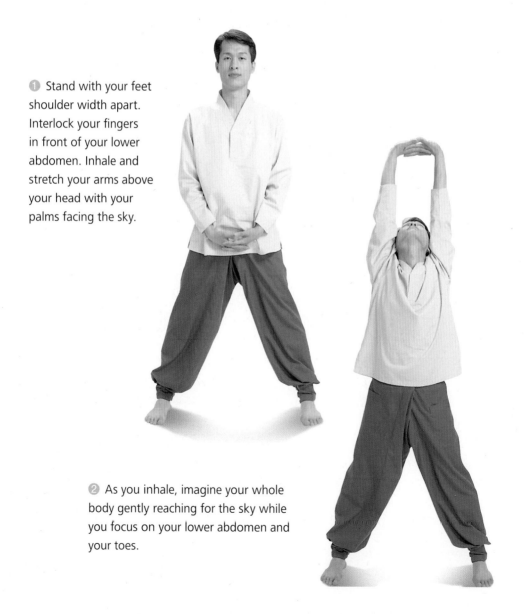

❶ Stand with your feet shoulder width apart. Interlock your fingers in front of your lower abdomen. Inhale and stretch your arms above your head with your palms facing the sky.

❷ As you inhale, imagine your whole body gently reaching for the sky while you focus on your lower abdomen and your toes.

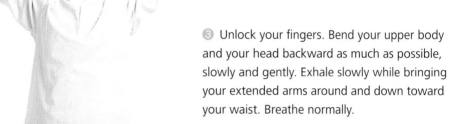

❸ Unlock your fingers. Bend your upper body and your head backward as much as possible, slowly and gently. Exhale slowly while bringing your extended arms around and down toward your waist. Breathe normally.

❹ Interlock your fingers at your lower abdomen again. Inhale and bend your upper body forward from your hips. Touch the floor with your palms.

❺ Exhale and return to STEP 1. Repeat the sequence 3 times.

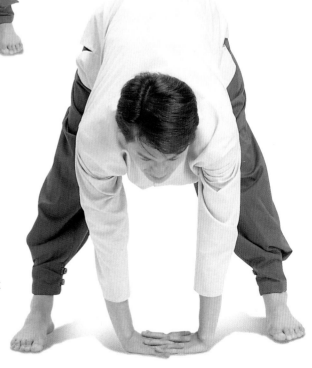

3. SWEEPING DOWN CHEST

BENEFITS Releases stagnant energy in the lungs and enhances blood circulation.

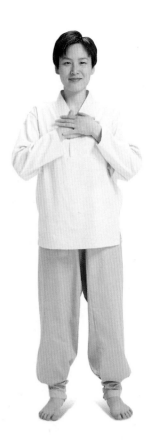

❶ Stand with your feet shoulder width apart and both hands resting on the center of your chest. Breathing slowly, deeply, and gently, methodically sweep your chest with downward strokes.

4. WRIST SHAKING

BENEFITS Releases stagnant energy from the Lung Meridian, strengthening the lungs and other organs.

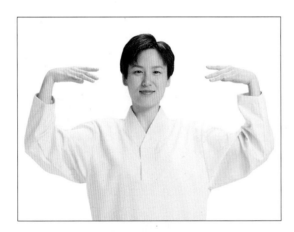

❶ Stand or sit with your chest open. Hold your arms to the sides at shoulder height with elbows bent at 90-degree angles and hands loosely held above the shoulders. Shake your wrists for a period from 30 seconds up to several minutes.

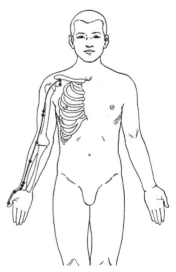

Lung Meridian
(extends from thumb up through shoulder to lung)

5. LUNG ENERGIZER

BENEFITS Strengthens the spinal cord and lungs, and brings fire energy that has accumulated in the lungs down to the lower abdomen. Expedites recovery from lung problems.

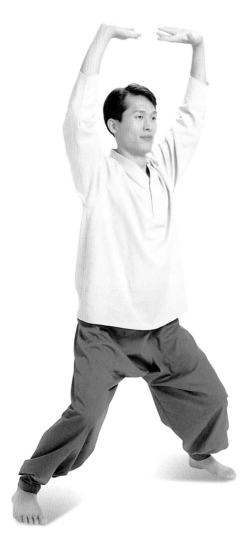

❶ Stand with your feet wider than shoulder width apart. Bring both of your arms above your head with your palms facing the sky and fingers pointing toward each other.

❷ Bend your knees slightly as you open your chest and lengthen your spine. Breathe normally. Hold this posture initially for 5 minutes. With increased practice, you can extend the time you hold this posture up to 30 minutes.

6. CHEST EXPANSION

BENEFITS Strengthens the heart and lungs while releasing excess fire energy. Decreases symptoms of blushing and hot flashes.

LUNG DISORDERS

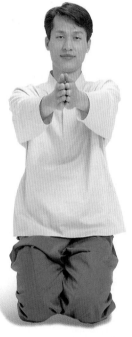

❶ Sit on your knees with buttocks resting on the heels and toes pointing forward. Extend your arms in front of you with your palms together. Inhale. Open your chest as you stretch your arms out to the sides with your palms facing forward.

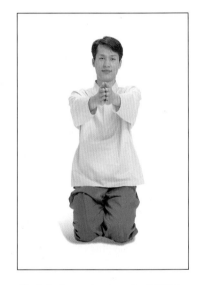

❷ Exhale and return to STEP 1.

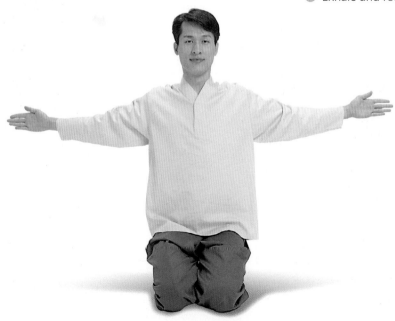

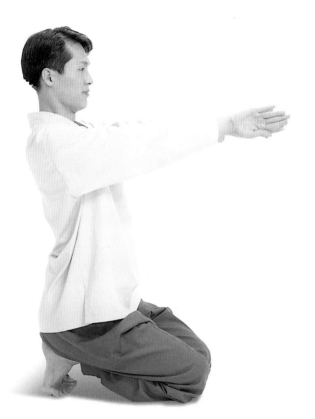

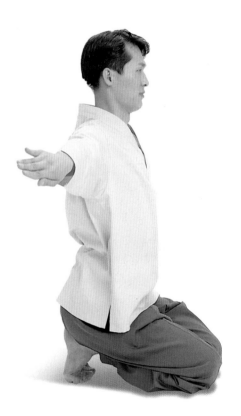

❸ Adjust your hands so the backs are touching and the palms are facing outward. Inhale and stretch your arms out to your sides with your palms facing behind you. Exhale and return your hands together.

❹ Move your hands so the palms are up and your pinkies are touching. Inhale and stretch your arms out to the sides with your palms up. Exhale and return your hands together.

❺ Turn your palms down with your thumbs touching. Inhale and stretch your arms out to your sides with your palms down. Exhale and return your hands together.

❻ The preceding STEPs compose one set of this exercise. Repeat the complete set 4 times.

7. ROTATING THE SHOULDERS

BENEFITS Relaxes the shoulders and facilitates blood circulation. Expands the chest to allow for symmetry and alignment of the spine and organs, so they can function at their maximum capacity.

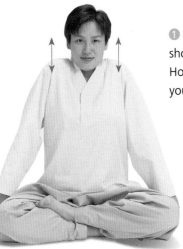

① While in the half-lotus position, raise your shoulders toward your ears as high as you can. Hold for a few seconds. Release the tension from your shoulders as you lower them.

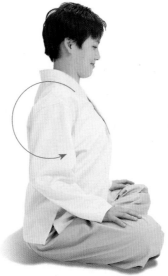

② Inhale while concentrating on your lower abdomen. Rotate your shoulders in forward circular motions. Repeat 5 times. Exhale.

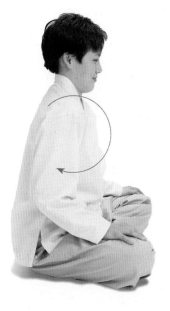

③ Inhale and rotate your shoulders in backward circular motions. Repeat 5 times. Exhale.

④ Repeat 3 times.

8. PULLING KNEE TOWARD THE CHEST

BENEFITS Facilitates blood circulation and lung respiration. Aligns the cervical spine.

TIPS When you pull your knee toward your chest, inhale, open your chest, and gently tense your arms, shoulders, waist, and lower abdomen. Simultaneously flex your opposite foot so toes are pointing toward you.

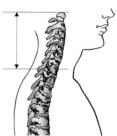

Cervical Vertebrae
Part of the spine from the base of the skull to the bottom of the neck.

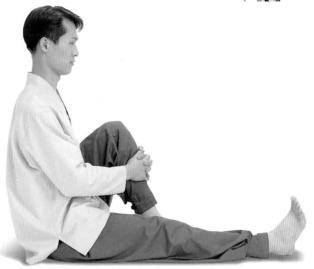

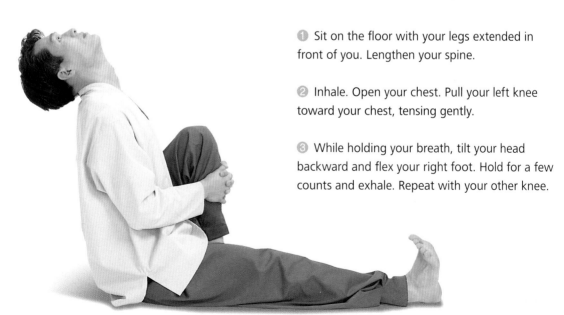

❶ Sit on the floor with your legs extended in front of you. Lengthen your spine.

❷ Inhale. Open your chest. Pull your left knee toward your chest, tensing gently.

❸ While holding your breath, tilt your head backward and flex your right foot. Hold for a few counts and exhale. Repeat with your other knee.

Respiratory System   *87*

COLDS AND FLU

Eastern Medicine adherents believe that when conditions in the environment are cold and damp, the energy produced by these factors can enter the body system, causing the person to feel ill with a cold or flu. Treatment consists of releasing the cold energy from the body.

The cold, moist energy initially enters through the acupressure point at the back of the neck, called the Poong-mun (Wind Gate, BL 12). Stimulating this point with massage and exercises will reduce cold and flu symptoms. It is imperative, particularly during the change of seasons, to ensure that warmth is maintained in these areas.

When you practice meridian exercise consistently, the immune system is boosted, thus thwarting the onset of colds and flus. If the system is compromised and one does come down with a cold or flu, the symptoms will be milder, and recovery will happen more quickly.

CLASPED HANDS FORWARD BEND (P. 79)

BENEFITS Assists in recovery from colds, cough, bronchitis, emphysema, and difficulty breathing.

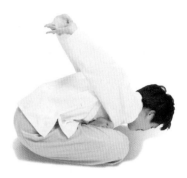

BACKWARD NECK TILT (P. 67)

BENEFITS Helps to open the energy channels around the neck and chest area.

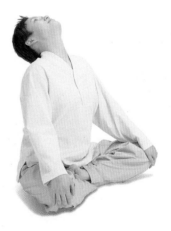

WHOLE BODY PATTING (P. 20)

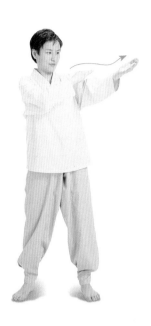

LUNG ENERGIZER (P. 83)

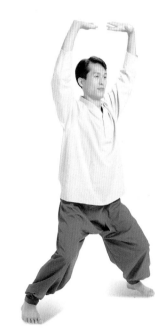

1. MASSAGE FOR COLD PREVENTION

BENEFITS Helps to clear cold congestion. Prevents or lessens duration of cold.

TIP Perform this exercise upon awakening in the morning.

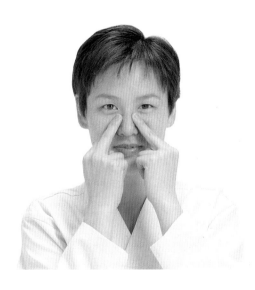

① Inhale. Place your fingers on either side of your nose, pressing and massaging the sinuses gently. Continue pressing under the eyes and along the eyebrows. Press and massage for about 5 minutes.

Respiratory System   *89*

2. TOE SQUATS

BENEFITS Boosts metabolism and the immune system, burns fat cells in the upper and lower body, and enhances blood and energy circulation.

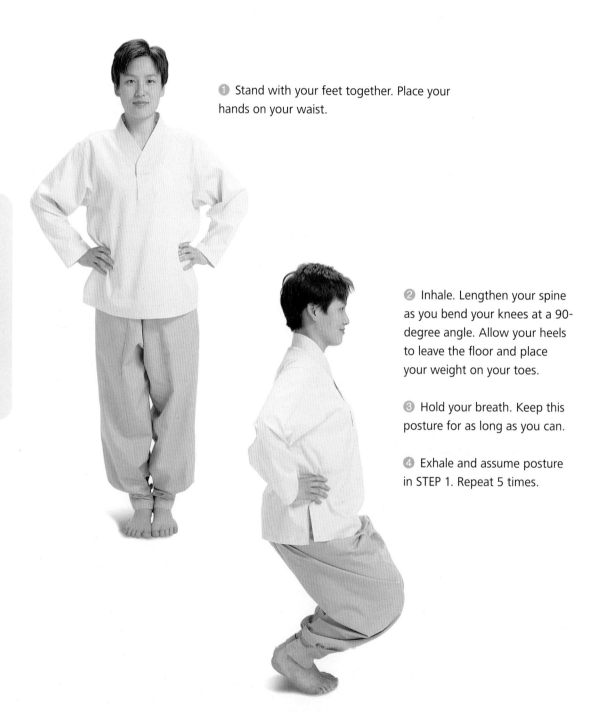

❶ Stand with your feet together. Place your hands on your waist.

❷ Inhale. Lengthen your spine as you bend your knees at a 90-degree angle. Allow your heels to leave the floor and place your weight on your toes.

❸ Hold your breath. Keep this posture for as long as you can.

❹ Exhale and assume posture in STEP 1. Repeat 5 times.

3. SHOULDER STRETCH

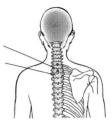

GV 14 (Dae-chu)
Second Thoracic Vertebra

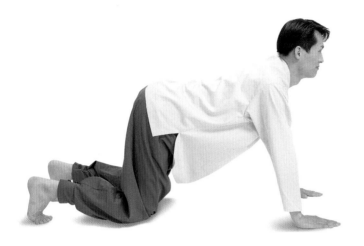

❶ Kneel on the floor with your knees at 90-degree angles and your palms on the floor below your shoulders. Bend your ankles with your toes pointed forward.

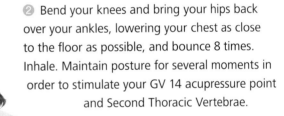

❷ Bend your knees and bring your hips back over your ankles, lowering your chest as close to the floor as possible, and bounce 8 times. Inhale. Maintain posture for several moments in order to stimulate your GV 14 acupressure point and Second Thoracic Vertebrae.

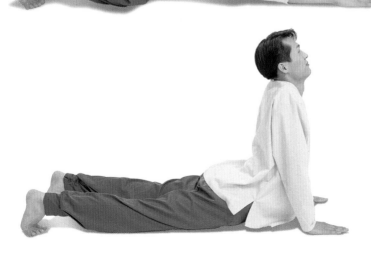

❸ Exhale. Keeping your toes on the floor, straighten your legs on the floor, moving your upper body forward. Arch your back and look toward the sky. Hold for 20-30 seconds and release. Repeat the whole procedure one more time.

4. SHOULDER DROP

TIPS When you inhale and raise your heels, tense your body. When you exhale, release all tension.

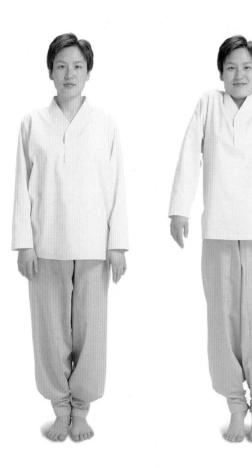

❶ Stand with your arms at your sides and feet together.

❷ Inhale. Raise your heels. Raise your shoulders toward your ears.

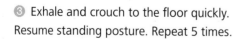

❸ Exhale and crouch to the floor quickly. Resume standing posture. Repeat 5 times.

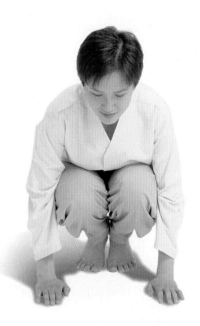

5. ARM EXTENSIONS

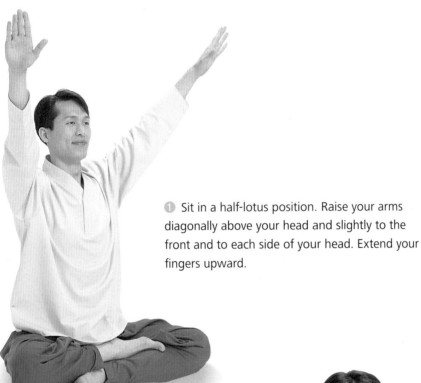

❶ Sit in a half-lotus position. Raise your arms diagonally above your head and slightly to the front and to each side of your head. Extend your fingers upward.

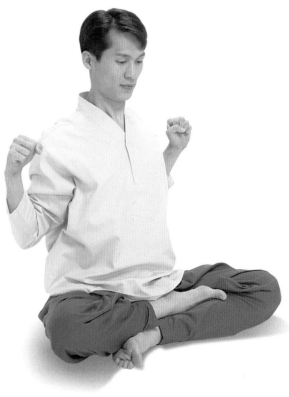

❷ Inhale. Make fists with your hands. Pull your fists down toward your shoulders, gently tensing your shoulder blades toward each other. Imagine you are pulling the oars of a rowboat.

❸ Exhale as you extend your arms to the STEP 1 position. Repeat 20 times.

6. HEAD TWIST

BENEFITS Regulates smooth Ki energy flow, enabling the release of cold energy from the GV 14 acupressure point.

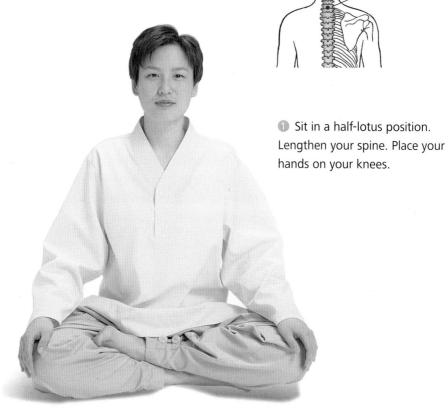

GV 14 (Dae-chu)

❶ Sit in a half-lotus position. Lengthen your spine. Place your hands on your knees.

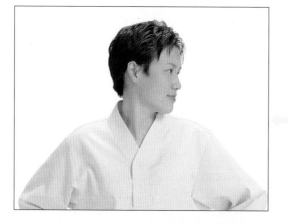

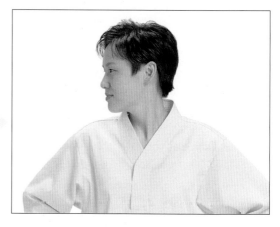

❷ Slowly turn your head to the right and left 30 times. Concentrate on the GV 14 acupressure point.

7. SHOULDERSTAND WITH WAIST SUPPORT

BENEFITS Maximizes Ki energy flow through the neck and brain, which helps to regulate the thyroid and to relieve headaches. Assists in lowering cholesterol, enhancing blood circulation, and detoxifying the blood throughout the body.

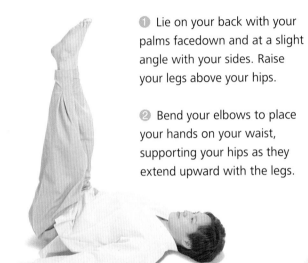

❶ Lie on your back with your palms facedown and at a slight angle with your sides. Raise your legs above your hips.

❷ Bend your elbows to place your hands on your waist, supporting your hips as they extend upward with the legs.

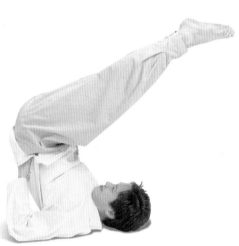

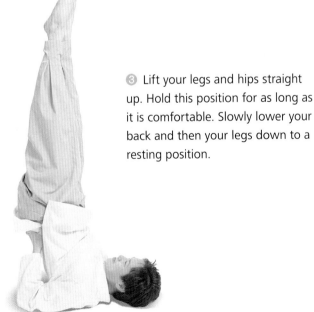

❸ Lift your legs and hips straight up. Hold this position for as long as it is comfortable. Slowly lower your back and then your legs down to a resting position.

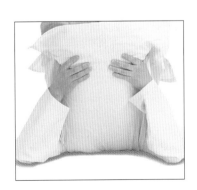

LOWER BACK PAIN

Lower back pain is a common malady. The etiology is multifaceted and may include faulty postural habits; lifting heavy objects improperly, fatigue, lack of sleep, and lack of exercise. Tension in the muscles located alongside the spine causes them to constrict, depriving them of oxygen. In order to thrive, muscles need purified oxygen transported throughout the blood so that the impulses in the nerves will activate correctly.

Tight hamstring muscles adversely affect the pelvis, thereby creating tension in muscles and tendons in the lower back. This, in turn, ultimately leads to misalignment of the spine, which may result in disk damage.

By performing meridian exercises regularly, the muscles will loosen and allow rich, oxygenated blood to flow into the muscles, nourishing them and permitting energy to circulate throughout the system. Relax your body to release tension. Then, very slowly begin to engage the meridian exercises recommended in this chapter, being mindful to perform only those which can be executed comfortably. It is best not to remain sedentary when afflicted with lower back pain because Ki energy can become obstructed, thus escalating the sensation and perception of pain and stiffness.

INTESTINE EXERCISE (P. 26)

BENEFITS Increases heat energy in the lower abdomen area, which permeates the body, including the lower back, spine, and organs.

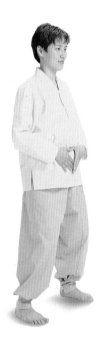

ABDOMINAL CLAPPING (P. 25)

BENEFITS Attracts Ki energy and blood circulation to your lower abdomen. It also strengthens the lower back area.

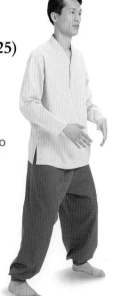

1. LEG SWEEP

BENEFITS This exercise increases heat energy in the lower abdomen area, which permeates the entire body, including the lower back, spine, and organs. It eases chronic lumbago and establishes an overall feeling of well-being.

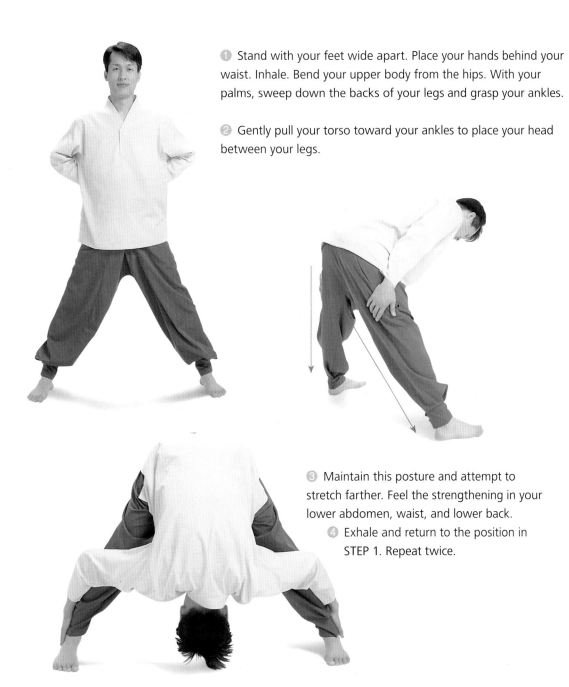

❶ Stand with your feet wide apart. Place your hands behind your waist. Inhale. Bend your upper body from the hips. With your palms, sweep down the backs of your legs and grasp your ankles.

❷ Gently pull your torso toward your ankles to place your head between your legs.

❸ Maintain this posture and attempt to stretch farther. Feel the strengthening in your lower abdomen, waist, and lower back.

❹ Exhale and return to the position in STEP 1. Repeat twice.

2. LYING HIP BOUNCE

BENEFITS Allows energy to circulate in the hips and waist, and strengthens organs.

TIP Relax your waist and lower extremities while performing this exercise.

LOWER BACK PAIN

❶ Lie on your back with your knees bent and your feet flat on the floor.

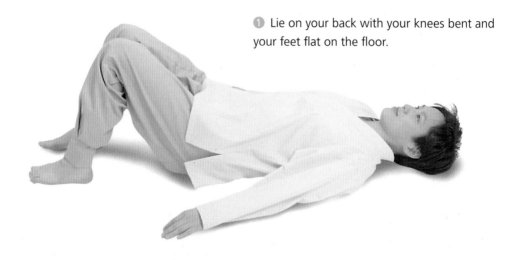

❷ Place your hands palms down on the floor, slightly away from your sides. Raise your hips and waist; then return them to the floor. Bounce your hips up and down for about 5 minutes. Extend the time as you continue to practice this exercise.

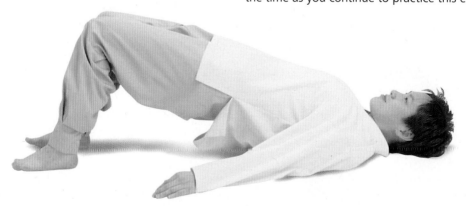

3. SIDE TO SIDE KNEES TWIST

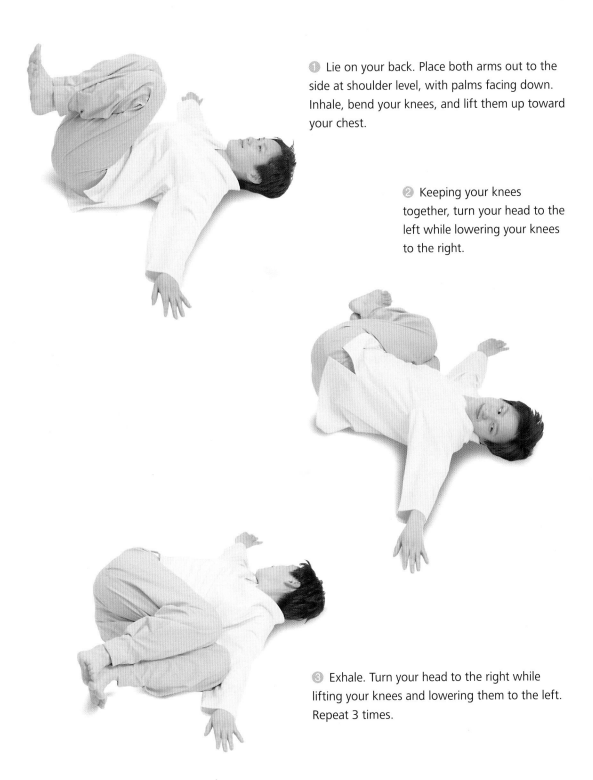

1 Lie on your back. Place both arms out to the side at shoulder level, with palms facing down. Inhale, bend your knees, and lift them up toward your chest.

2 Keeping your knees together, turn your head to the left while lowering your knees to the right.

3 Exhale. Turn your head to the right while lifting your knees and lowering them to the left. Repeat 3 times.

4. PELVIS REALIGNMENT

TIPS To perform this exercise correctly, it is necessary to twist your upper body in the opposite direction of your lower body.

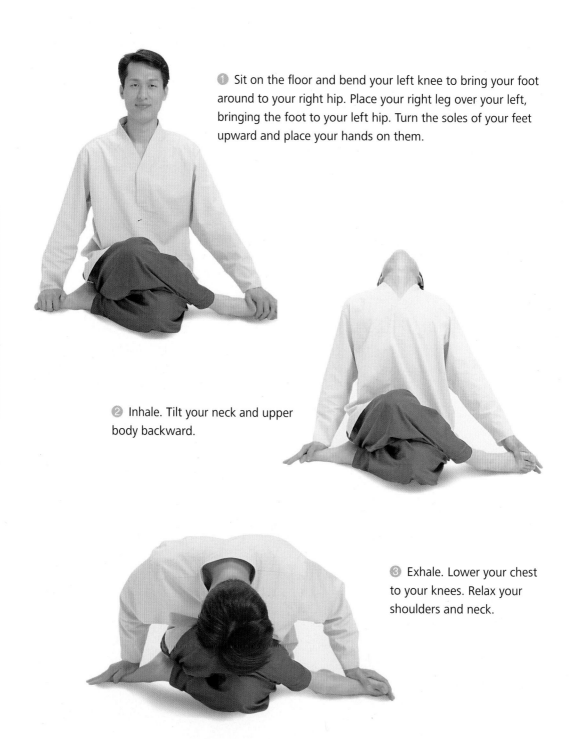

① Sit on the floor and bend your left knee to bring your foot around to your right hip. Place your right leg over your left, bringing the foot to your left hip. Turn the soles of your feet upward and place your hands on them.

② Inhale. Tilt your neck and upper body backward.

③ Exhale. Lower your chest to your knees. Relax your shoulders and neck.

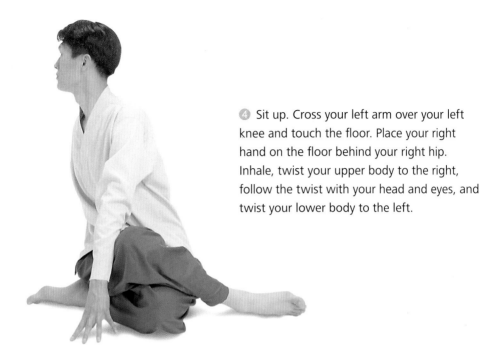

④ Sit up. Cross your left arm over your left knee and touch the floor. Place your right hand on the floor behind your right hip. Inhale, twist your upper body to the right, follow the twist with your head and eyes, and twist your lower body to the left.

⑤ Exhale. Return to STEP 1. Repeat twice. Switch the positions of your legs and twist to the opposite side.

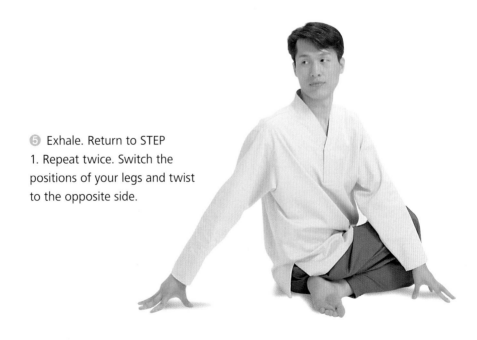

5. FACE-DOWN TOE TOUCH

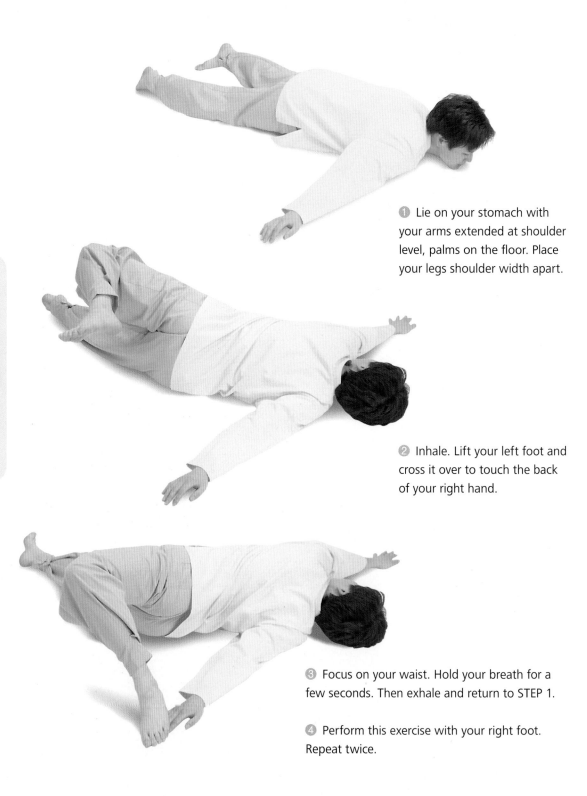

❶ Lie on your stomach with your arms extended at shoulder level, palms on the floor. Place your legs shoulder width apart.

❷ Inhale. Lift your left foot and cross it over to touch the back of your right hand.

❸ Focus on your waist. Hold your breath for a few seconds. Then exhale and return to STEP 1.

❹ Perform this exercise with your right foot. Repeat twice.

6. LYING LOTUS STRETCH

BENEFITS Aligns and strengthens the lumbar spine and opens the chest.

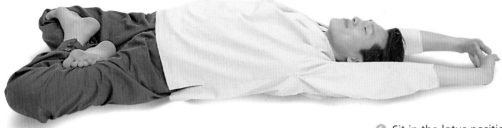

❶ Sit in the lotus position and lie back. Stretch your arms above your head and interlace your fingers.

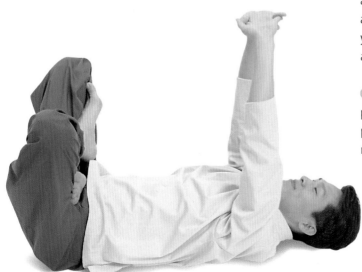

❷ Simultaneously lift your legs above your hips and your arms above your shoulders. Relax your arms and legs to the floor again.

❸ Repeat 15 times. Switch the position of your legs in the lotus position and then repeat 15 more times.

7. WAGGING YOUR FEET

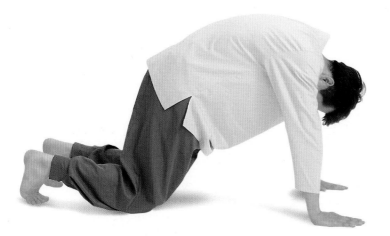

❶ Kneel on the floor with your hips above your knees and your palms on the floor below your shoulders. Bend your ankles with your toes pointing forward. Inhale. Round your back upward and bend your neck downward.

❷ Exhale. Lower your waist. Bring your head up. Repeat 5 times.

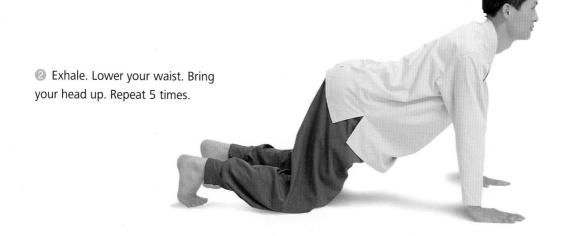

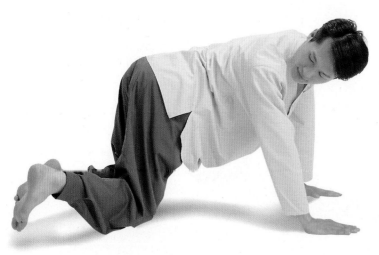

❸ Bring your feet off the floor and twist them out to one side, following the movement with your head and eyes. Switch sides. Perform as many times as you like.

8. PULLING KNEES TO CHEST

TIP Do not perform this exercise if you have been diagnosed with high blood pressure.

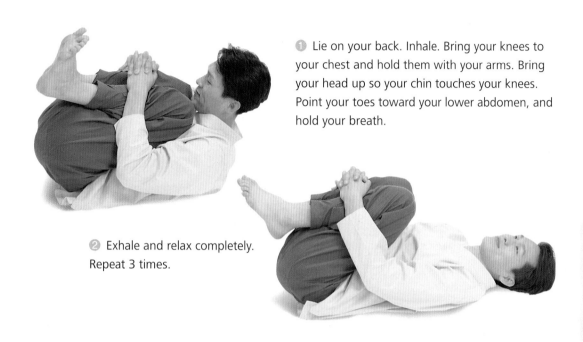

① Lie on your back. Inhale. Bring your knees to your chest and hold them with your arms. Bring your head up so your chin touches your knees. Point your toes toward your lower abdomen, and hold your breath.

② Exhale and relax completely. Repeat 3 times.

9. UPPER BODY LIFT

BENEFITS Exercises 9 and 10 strengthen your upper abdomen and waist, and realign the lumbar spine.

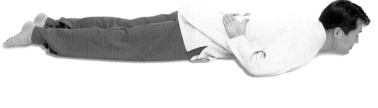

① Lie on your stomach with your legs together. Place your hands palms up on the back of your waist.

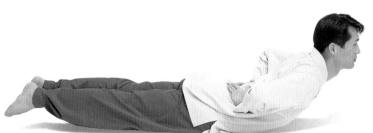

② Arch your back to lift your torso. Simultaneously lift your feet and point your toes.

③ Return to STEP 1. Repeat 20 times.

10. SIT-UP

TIPS Perform this exercise very slowly. Pay attention to the sensations in your waist and abdomen.

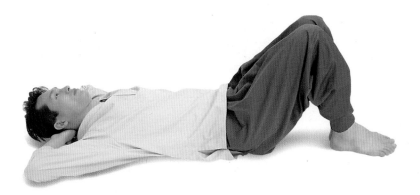

❶ Have a partner hold your legs in place, or place your legs under a surface where they will be supported and stationary.

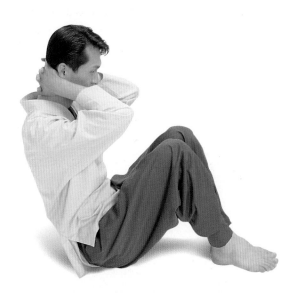

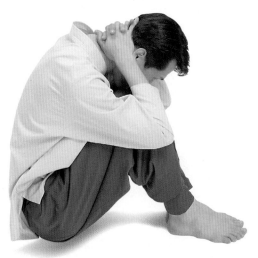

❷ Lie on your back with your knees bent and feet flat on the floor. Interlock your fingers behind your neck.

❸ Raise your upper body and attempt to touch your knees with your elbows. Repeat according to your physical condition.

11. SLEEPING TIGER ENERGIZER

BENEFITS Relieves lumbago and stimulates the kidneys. Expedites Ki energy accumulation in the lower abdomen, strengthens muscles around the waist, and relieves pain in the neck and the shoulders.

TIPS If you have been diagnosed with disk problems, perform this exercise carefully. Cautiously increase the time you maintain this posture.

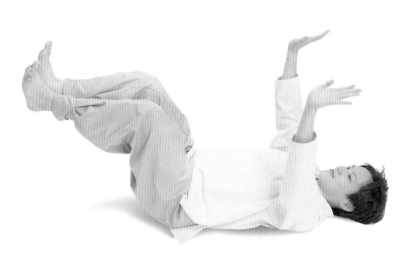

❶ Lie on your back. Bring your arms straight above your shoulders with your wrists bent and palms up. Bring your knees up so they are almost directly above your hips and flex your feet. Relax your neck and shoulders and the rest of your body. Breathe naturally.

❷ Focus on your lower abdomen. Hold this pose for as long as it is comfortable.

❸ As you begin practicing this exercise, let your head relax on the floor. As you increase your practice time, lift your head while performing this posture.

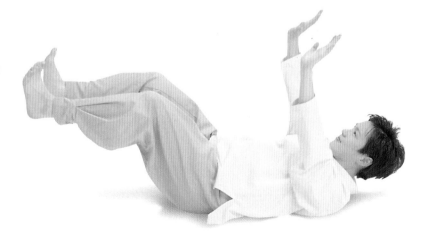

NECK PAIN

The seven vertebrae of the cervical spine compose the neck, which connects the head and body with nervous system activity. Muscles surrounding the neck keep it erect.

When you experience pain in the neck area, the cause is most commonly muscular problems. Sometimes there may be a herniated or protruding disk. One of the ways to detect a disk problem is to sit in the lotus position. Place your palms on top of your head and push down on the head. If you experience pain, it may signal a disk problem. Cervical misalignment or stiffness of muscles around the neck and shoulders could also be accompanied by neck pain.

If you have a diagnosed disk problem, observe yourself. Relax your neck and shoulders, and rotate your neck in different positions, watching how your neck moves. Choose from the postures here to find those that serve your particular condition best.

If you have a protruding or herniated disk in your cervical or lumbar spine, it could signal a problem in the liver or kidneys. These exercises will help to stimulate and challenge the liver, kidneys, and cervical spine. If you experience neck pain, it is imperative to keep the neck warm with a hot compress for twenty minutes at a time.

NECK MASSAGE (P. 35)

TIP When you massage your neck, you can focus on the areas where you have pain.

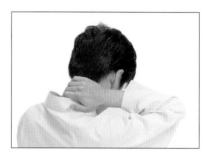

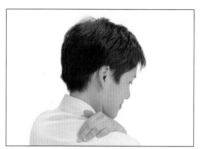

MOVING A JAR (P. 47)

BENEFITS Aligns the spine and rib cage. Helps to relieve cervical disk problems, facial paralysis, shoulder pain, and symptoms of tuberculosis.

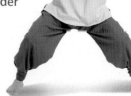

SLEEPING TIGER ENERGIZER (P. 107)

BENEFITS If you raise your head, circulation in the head and neck is more efficient, relieving neck pain. This exercise also aligns the cervical spine and strengthens neck muscles.

TIPS If you have a diagnosed problem in your cervical spine, you may wish to proceed with this posture by keeping your head on the floor. Exercise caution and judgment with this position.

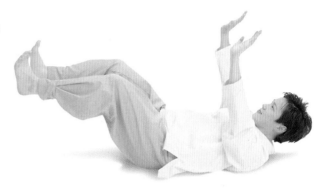

1. USING A WOODEN PILLOW

BENEFITS This exercise expedites energy flow to the head, brain, and nervous system. It enhances mental clarity and visual acuity. It also opens acupressure points around the neck and aligns the spinal cord.

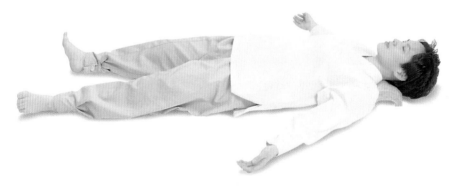

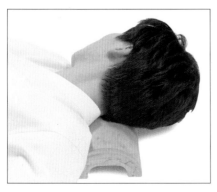

❶ Lie on your back with the wooden pillow under your neck, resting your head. Relax. Turn your head slowly so your ear touches the wooden pillow. Slowly turn to the other side.

❷ If you experience pain while performing this, your neck muscles may be stiff. If you are pain free during this exercise, you can consider using the wooden pillow while you sleep.

2. HEAD LIFT

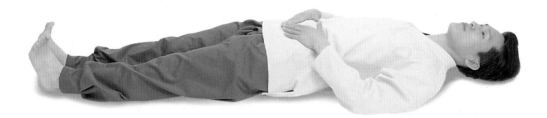

1 Lie down on your back with your legs extended, feet together, and your toes flexed toward your body. Place your hands on your lower abdomen with your thumbs and index fingers touching, forming a triangle.

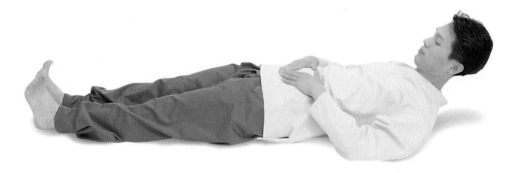

2 Lift your head slowly and gradually lower it again, but do not let it touch the floor.

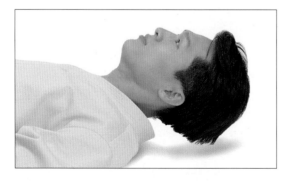 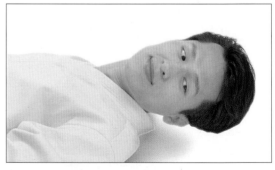

3 Continue to move your head up and down, slowly and carefully. Alternate turning your head left and right as you lift it. Repeat the motion 20 times.

3. NECK EXERCISE

TIPS Focus on your neck. Very slowly, move only your neck and head. Relax the rest of your body.

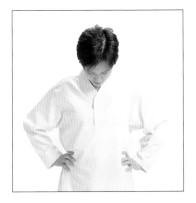 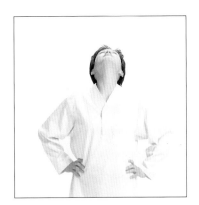

① Stand with your hands on your waist. Drop your head forward so your chin touches your chest. Move your head very slowly in a circular motion. Breathe naturally.

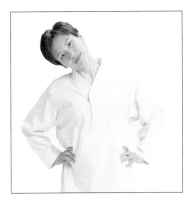 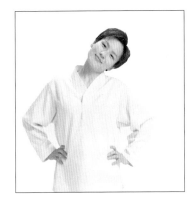

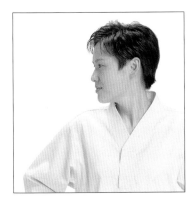

② Inhale. Slowly turn your head to the left. Hold your breath. Face forward again and exhale through your mouth. As you do this, imagine the stagnant energy from your neck exiting the body through your mouth. Repeat this movement to the right.

NECK PAIN

BONE, MUSCLE, AND SKIN

SHOULDER PAIN

Pain in the shoulders is most often caused by stress. When you experience stress or high blood pressure, for example, the shoulder muscles can spasm or stiffen. Pain in the shoulder region may also be caused by organ malfunction or poor postural habits.

The shoulder is the conduit for blood circulation into the brain. When the muscles in the shoulder contract, oxygen in the blood cannot pass easily to the brain, thereby depriving the brain.

Consequently, functions of the major organs, such as the lungs and heart, are compromised. In Eastern Medicine, it is believed that when shoulder pain is present, blood becomes stagnant and energy is blocked around the muscles of the neck and shoulder. As the problem persists, the range of motion in the shoulder decreases while the pain intensifies.

The exercises recommended in this chapter can ultimately bring significant relief from shoulder pain. This is because the exercises provide improved Ki energy and blood circulation, with fresh oxygen flow to nourish the muscles and to release stagnant blood from the affected shoulder area.

NECK MASSAGE (P. 35)

TIP In addition to self-massage, you can also ask someone to assist you in massaging the painful muscle area in the back of your neck.

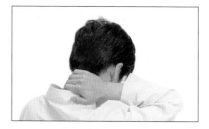

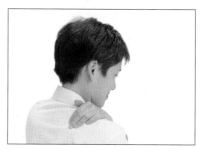

CLASPED HANDS FORWARD BEND (P. 79)

BENEFITS Expands chest to enhance and strengthen blood circulation in the lungs and endocrine system. Speeds the process through which your body releases toxins.

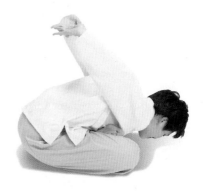

112 Meridian Exercise

1. PUSHING PALMS

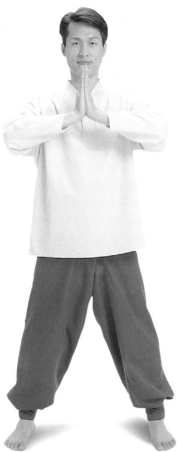

1 Stand with your feet shoulder width apart and your palms together in front of your chest. Inhale. Hold your breath while you open your chest and press your palms together. Hold for a few seconds. Exhale and relax. Repeat f5 times.

2. PULLING THE ELBOW BEHIND THE HEAD

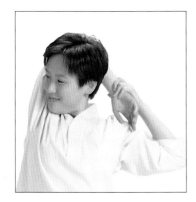
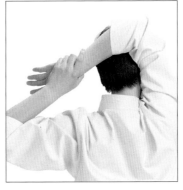
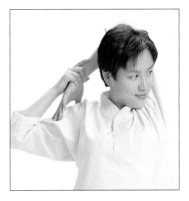

1 Place your right arm behind your head, elbow bent. Hold your right wrist with your left hand. Inhale. Pull gently on your right wrist while focusing on your shoulder joint.

2 Exhale. Release. Repeat twice with each arm.

3. CROSS ARMS, CLASP, AND TWIST

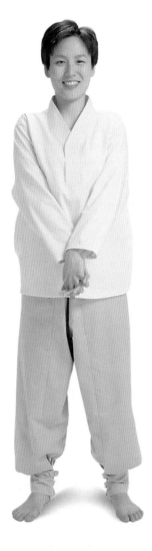

❶ Cross your wrists, bring your palms together, and interlace your fingers. Inhale. Bend your elbows to bring your hands under your arms and toward your chest in a circular motion. Continue the motion to extend your arms in front of your chest. Continuing to clasp your hands, tilt your head backward and stretch.

❷ Hold for a few seconds. Exhale. Return to STEP 1 and switch the position of your hands to repeat the exercise.

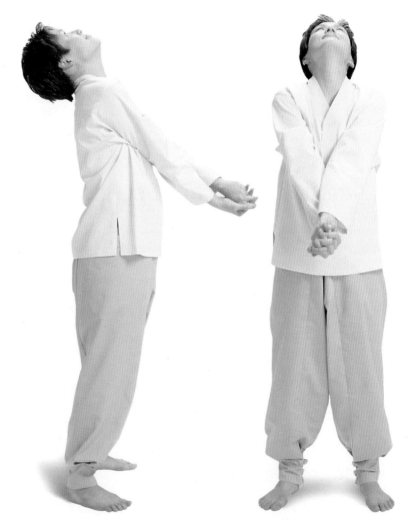

4. ARM ROTATIONS

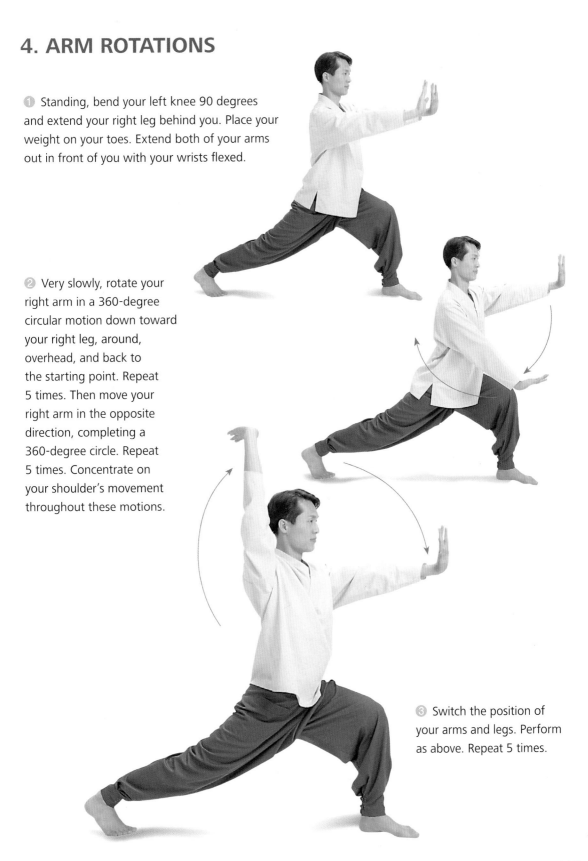

❶ Standing, bend your left knee 90 degrees and extend your right leg behind you. Place your weight on your toes. Extend both of your arms out in front of you with your wrists flexed.

❷ Very slowly, rotate your right arm in a 360-degree circular motion down toward your right leg, around, overhead, and back to the starting point. Repeat 5 times. Then move your right arm in the opposite direction, completing a 360-degree circle. Repeat 5 times. Concentrate on your shoulder's movement throughout these motions.

❸ Switch the position of your arms and legs. Perform as above. Repeat 5 times.

5. UPPER BODY BEND WITH SHOULDER STRETCH

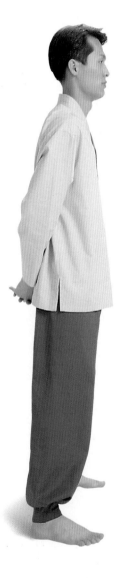

❶ Stand with your legs shoulder width apart. Clasp your hands behind your back, palms facing upward.

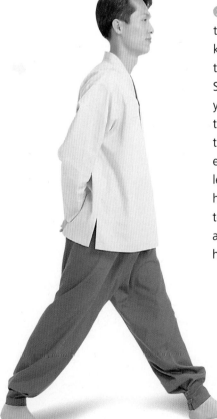

❷ Inhale. Turn your body to the left. Bend your right knee. Turn your right foot to the left at a 45-degree angle. Straighten your left knee with your heel on the floor and your toes pointing upward. Bend at the hips so your upper body extends down over the left leg while you lift your clasped hands upward behind your back to a comfortable height. Look at your toes as you bend your head down toward your knee.

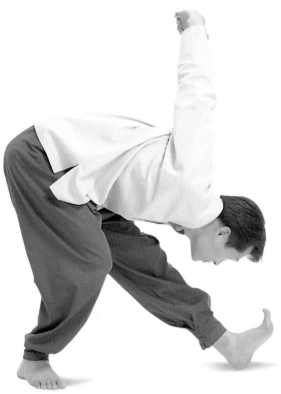

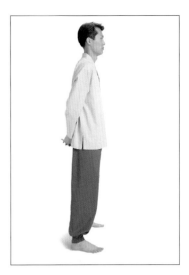

❸ Exhale. Return to STEP 1. Perform this exercise with your opposite leg.

❹ Place your feet together. Inhale. Bend your trunk forward, moving your face toward your knees, and raise your clasped hands comfortably behind your back.

❺ Exhale and stand up. Repeat each side 2 times.

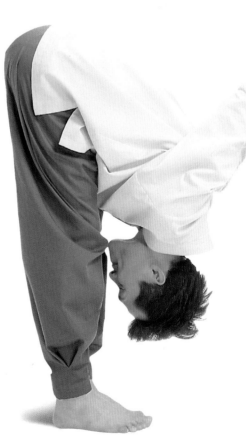

6. HAND CLAPPING

BENEFITS Brings heat energy around the shoulder muscles as Ki energy and blood circulation are facilitated.

❶ Stand with your feet shoulder width apart. Touch your palms together about a foot in front of your face.

❷ Clap your hands in front of your face, behind your head, and behind your waist, one time each. This completes one repetition. Keep your head straight while relaxing the muscles in your neck and shoulders. Repeat 50 times.

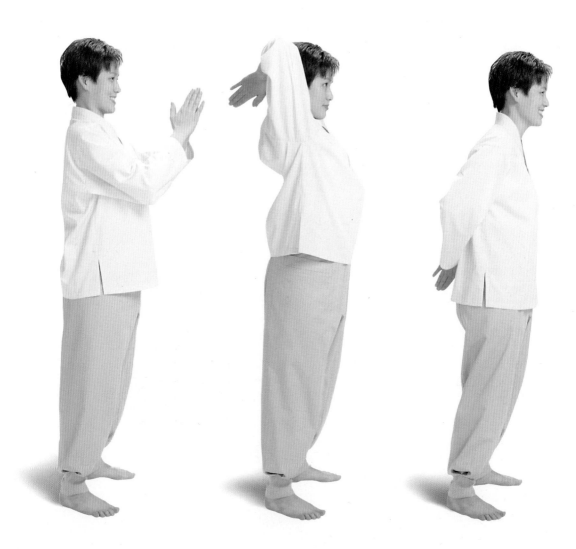

7. FORWARD SHOULDER STRETCH

BENEFITS Relieves tension in the shoulder muscles, hands, and arms. Rejuvenates the hand as you stimulate the meridians on the back of your hand.

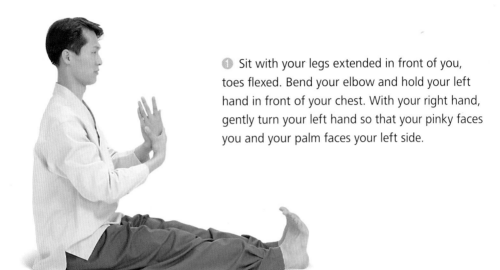

1 Sit with your legs extended in front of you, toes flexed. Bend your elbow and hold your left hand in front of your chest. With your right hand, gently turn your left hand so that your pinky faces you and your palm faces your left side.

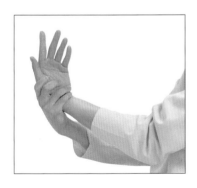

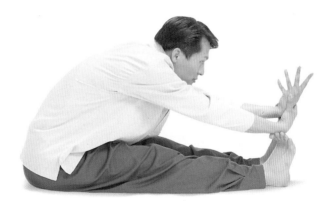

2 Place the four fingers of your right hand on the pad of your left palm. Place your right thumb about halfway up the back of the left hand between the ring and pinky fingers. Slightly twist your left hand as you press into the back of your left hand with your right thumb. This acupressure position will activate several meridians.

3 Inhale. While maintaining the position of your hands, bend your trunk forward, with your arms extended, to touch your toes with the back of your right hand. Focus on your shoulders. Exhale and return to STEP 1. Repeat with the opposite hand.

SCIATIC PAIN

The sciatic nerve, which originates in the lumbar spine and runs down the legs, is the largest of the peripheral nerves. Sciatic pain, known as sciatica, is considered severe by most people who experience it. The pain radiates deeply into the muscles of the buttocks, coursing down the posterior part of each leg and through the back of the thigh and calf. In severe cases, pain extends into the foot. It can be accompanied by numbness and tingling.

The causes of sciatica can be multifaceted, including peripheral nerve root compression from herniated disks, weakness of the kidneys, poor posture habits, and long-term sedentary lifestyle, or changes in joints due to bony growths, such as osteoarthritis, muscle spasms, or irritated tissues around the joints of the spine. In severe cases, people compensate for the pain by shifting their weight into other parts of their body—often favoring the side of the body free from sciatica—causing misalignment and exacerbating the problem.

It is important to maintain warmth in the lower part of the body when you experience sciatic nerve difficulty.

CLASPED HANDS FORWARD BEND (P. 79)

TIPS If you can, sit in a half-lotus position to perform this exercise. If you cannot assume this position, then perform with your legs crossed.

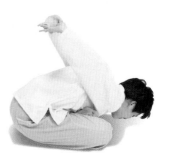

CROSSING LEGS AND TWISTING (P. 77)

BENEFITS Relaxes knee joints, allows maximum proficiency of the autonomic nervous system, and regulates intestines and accompanying organs. Promotes flexibility of the lower extremities and prevents or helps to abate neuralgia.

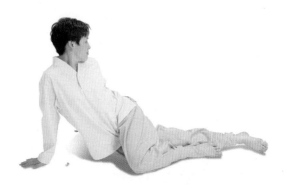

1. FOOT TO THIGH FORWARD BEND

TIPS Do not strain to touch your toes. Instead, reach forward as far as is most comfortably challenging.

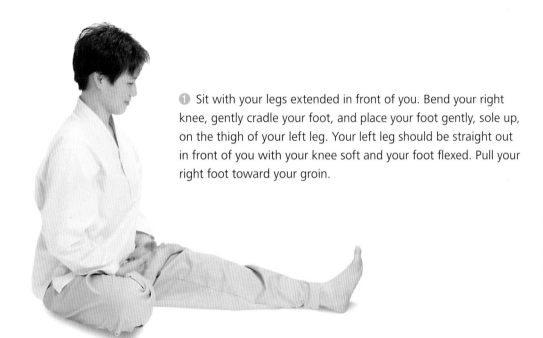

❶ Sit with your legs extended in front of you. Bend your right knee, gently cradle your foot, and place your foot gently, sole up, on the thigh of your left leg. Your left leg should be straight out in front of you with your knee soft and your foot flexed. Pull your right foot toward your groin.

❷ Bend forward from your hips. Reach both hands toward your left foot and, if comfortable, grasp your left foot. Bend your torso gently toward your left knee.

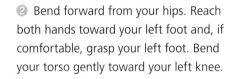

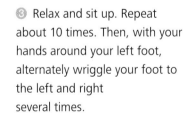

❸ Relax and sit up. Repeat about 10 times. Then, with your hands around your left foot, alternately wriggle your foot to the left and right several times.

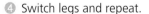

❹ Switch legs and repeat.

2. REACH, TWIST, AND BEND

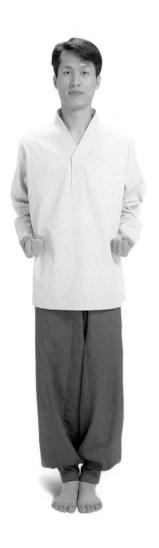

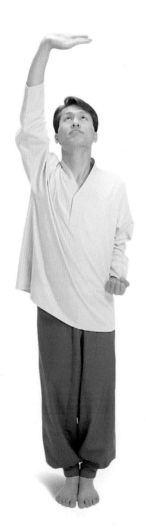

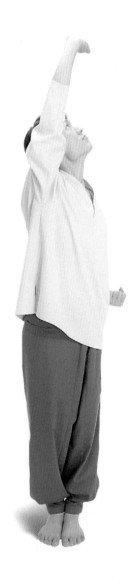

● Stand with your feet touching together. Place your hands, palms up, at your sides and close them into firm fists.

● Inhale. Raise your right hand toward the sky. Open it so the palm faces up and your elbow is slightly bent, pointing to the side. Follow this movement of your hand with your head and eyes.

● Hold your breath. Twist your upper body to the left.

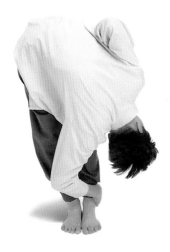

④ Bend slowly from your hips. Grasp your left ankle with your right hand. Keep your knees straight but relaxed. Focus on your lower abdomen and lower back.

⑤ Exhale. Return to STEP 1 and perform to the opposite side. Repeat 3 times on each side.

3. FORWARD BUTTERFLY BEND

BENEFITS This exercise promotes maximum Ki energy flow to the abdominal area, calms the mind, and rejuvenates the skin. It helps to prevent or abate neuralgia and promotes flexibility in the knee joints.

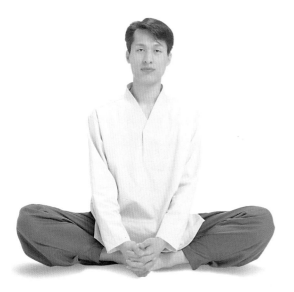

① Sit with your knees bent and the soles of your feet touching. Gently and comfortably pull your feet in toward your groin as much as possible. Cup your feet with your hands, releasing any tension in your hands.

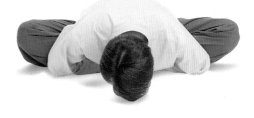

② Inhale. Keeping your spine straight, bend forward from your hips. Bend down as far as you comfortably can. Focus on your waist and your hip joints, and hold for several seconds. With practice, you may be able to touch your forehead to the floor.

③ Exhale and return to STEP 1. Repeat motion 3 times.

4. EXTENDED LEG TO TOE TOUCH

❶ Sit with your right leg straight out in front of you. Bend your left knee and bring your left foot to rest next to your right thigh. Place your hands in a prayer position in front of your chest.

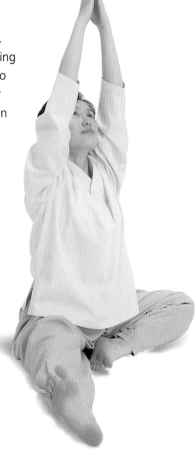

❷ Inhale. Raise your arms straight up above your head with your palms touching. Follow the movement with your eyes.

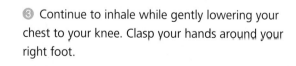

❸ Continue to inhale while gently lowering your chest to your knee. Clasp your hands around your right foot.

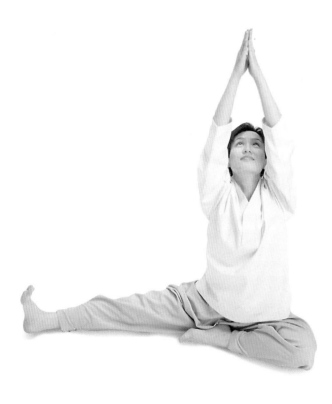

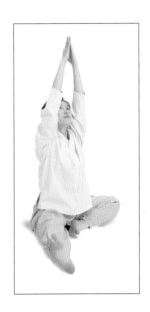

④ Exhale and return to STEP 1.

⑤ Inhale. Raise your palms together above your head.

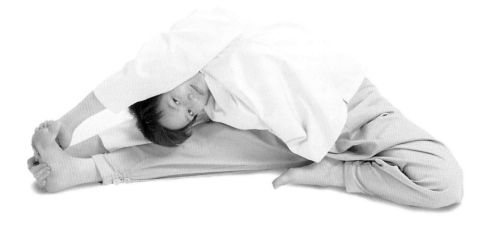

⑥ Continue to inhale. Lean to the right and bend your right side over your extended leg. Look upward as you touch your knee with your head. Wrap your hands around your right foot.

⑦ Exhale. Return to STEP 1. Switch legs and repeat.

5. INNER THIGH STRETCH

BENEFITS Enhances nervous system functioning in the waist, legs, and hip joints. Alleviates pain in the lower back.

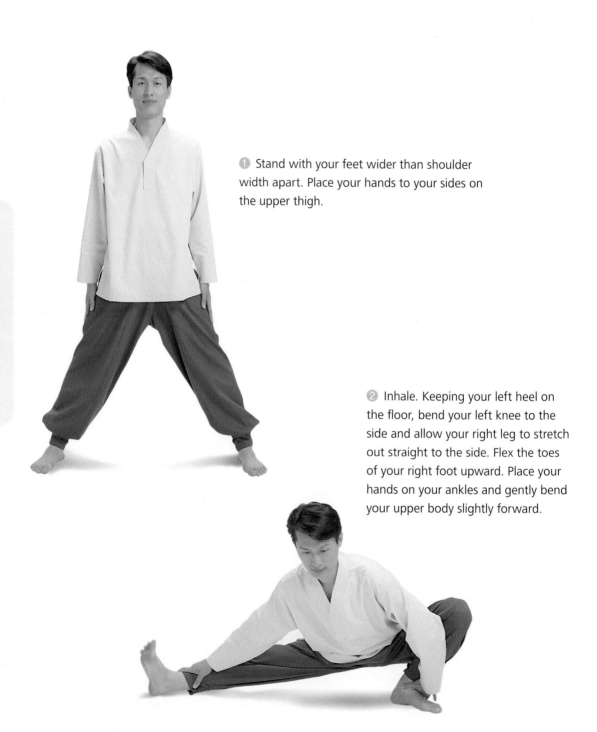

❶ Stand with your feet wider than shoulder width apart. Place your hands to your sides on the upper thigh.

❷ Inhale. Keeping your left heel on the floor, bend your left knee to the side and allow your right leg to stretch out straight to the side. Flex the toes of your right foot upward. Place your hands on your ankles and gently bend your upper body slightly forward.

③ Continue inhaling and bending your upper body. Turn your upper body toward your right leg, and bend your forehead toward your right knee.

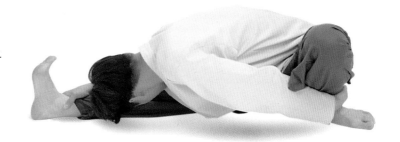

④ Exhale. Return to STEP 1. Repeat to the opposite side.

⑤ From STEP 1, turn to the left and swivel your feet so the left toes point forward. Place the right toes at a 45-degree angle. Bend your left knee 90 degrees so your right leg extends behind you, and place your left hand on your left thigh. Place your right hand on the back of your right thigh.

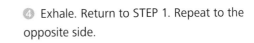

⑥ Inhale, open your chest, and tilt your head back as you raise your right heel off the floor, keeping your right leg straight. Focus on your thighs and calves.

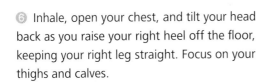

ARTHRITIS

The term *arthritis* technically refers to joint inflammation. While there are several types of arthritis, this chapter will describe the two most prevalent forms: rheumatoid and degenerative arthritis. Rheumatoid arthritis is the most frequently diagnosed incapacitating form of arthritis. It is an autoimmune disease caused by the immune system launching an assault upon the joints, causing inflammation, stiffness, pain, redness, swelling, and heat. Due to toxins that accumulate as a result of prolonged inflammation, rheumatoid arthritis can also affect organs and muscles.

Degenerative joint disease, or osteoarthritis, is a form of arthritis usually associated with aging. Those with this disease experience stiffness and decreased range of motion. This disease occurs as the tissue between the bones in joints, known as the articular cartilage, deteriorates. Bony growths can occur with hard nodules, which differ from the more spongy inflammation in the joints of someone with rheumatoid arthritis. Knees and hips are frequently attacked by degenerative joint disease because of the weight these joints must bear.

The six major joints, including the elbows, wrists, knees, hips, and ankles, are the most vulnerable targets for arthritis and the prime locations where energy is blocked. Ki energy and blood circulation in these joints become compromised and restricted.

Unfortunately, when a person experiences pain from the inflammation of arthritis, the natural tendency is to avoid movement, which creates a vicious cycle, immobilizing the joint and further limiting its function. To restore movement, energy blockages must be released to re-enable function. Ki energy and blood circulation must be augmented.

The exercises in this chapter are designed to promote this process. As with any other diagnosed condition discussed in this book, consult a health care professional for additional advice.

Meridian exercises can help to manage the sensation of pain due to arthritis. Progressive deterioration of the joints can be deterred. As Ki energy and blood circulation freely move throughout your system, flexibility and strength of muscles and ligaments can be refined, increasing range of motion and protecting joints. Impact on joints is significantly minimized and a sense of well-being is experienced as you synchronize conscious breathing with your body's movements.

PUSH AND PULL TOE GRAB (P. 73)

BENEFITS Stimulates the kidneys and joints, including knee joints, and helps to alleviate shoulder pain.

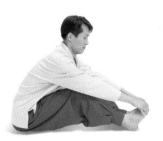

1. HAMSTRING MUSCLE RELEASE

BENEFITS Releases stagnant Ki energy from behind the knees. Ki and blood circulation are facilitated and knee joints are nourished.

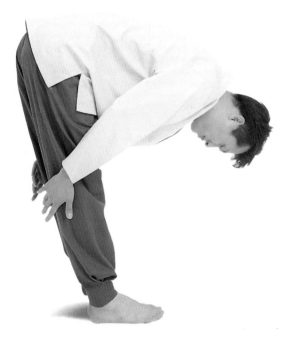

❶ Stand with your feet together. Bend at the hips and use your hands to pat and massage the backs of your knees continuously.

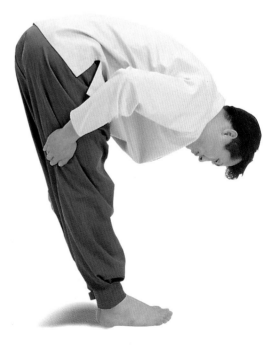

❷ Then sweep repeatedly down the backs of your legs with your palms to release stagnant energy.

2. KNEE FLEXION AND EXTENSION

TIPS When you exhale, imagine that you are releasing stagnant energy from your knees and sending it out through your toes.

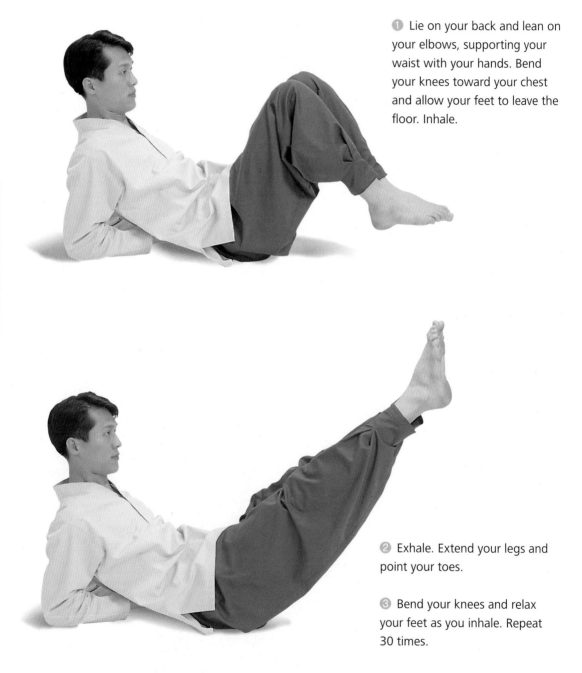

❶ Lie on your back and lean on your elbows, supporting your waist with your hands. Bend your knees toward your chest and allow your feet to leave the floor. Inhale.

❷ Exhale. Extend your legs and point your toes.

❸ Bend your knees and relax your feet as you inhale. Repeat 30 times.

3. KNEE MASSAGE

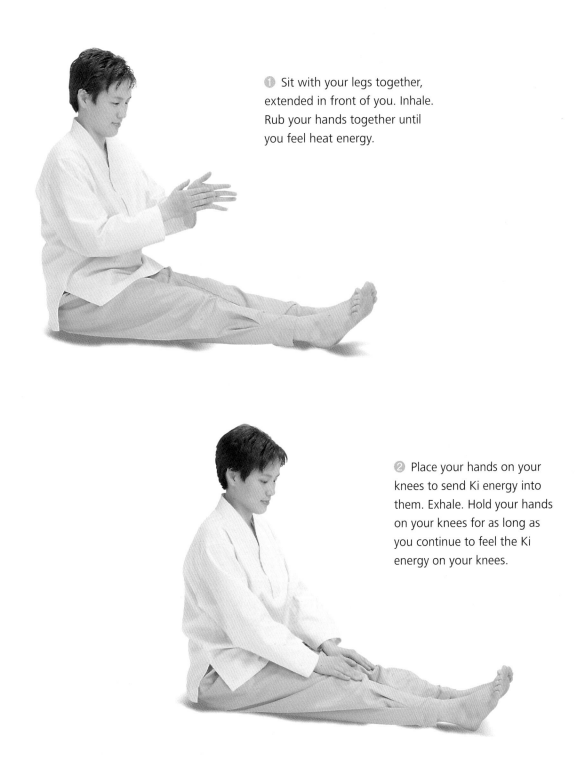

1 Sit with your legs together, extended in front of you. Inhale. Rub your hands together until you feel heat energy.

2 Place your hands on your knees to send Ki energy into them. Exhale. Hold your hands on your knees for as long as you continue to feel the Ki energy on your knees.

4. KNEE EXERCISE

TIPS Keep your back relaxed and elongated and your feet parallel to your shoulders. Increase the length of time you hold the pose as you progress in your practice.

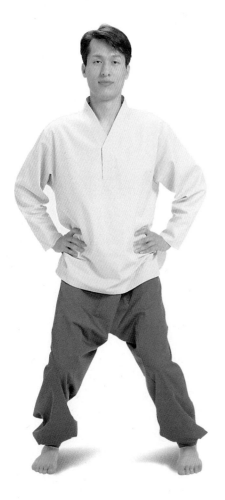

❶ Stand with your feet shoulder width apart. Place your hands on your waist. Keep your spine relaxed and elongated, not stiff. Inhale. Bend your knees about 15 degrees.

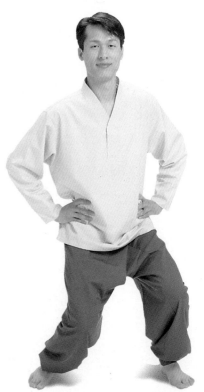

❷ Hold your breath. Rotate your knees slowly to the left. Return to facing forward. Repeat the rotations 3 times.

❸ Then rotate your knees to the right 3 times. Repeat this sequence 5 times. Focus on your knees becoming warmer.

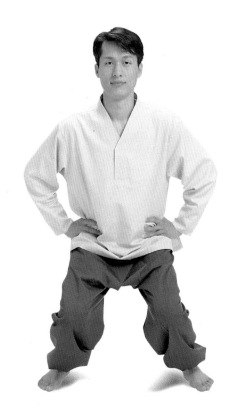

④ Inhale. Bend your knees as much as possible while keeping your spine relaxed and back straight. Exhale and return to standing position. Repeat 15 times.

5. JOINT ENERGIZER

BENEFITS Attracts heat to knees, relaxes hip joints, and releases stagnant energy from lower extremities. Facilitates Ki energy and blood circulation of lower extremities.

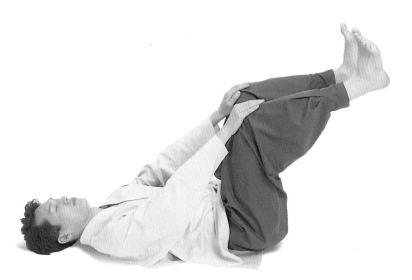

Lie down on your back. Raise your knees above your hips and flex your toes. Place both hands on your knees, as demonstrated in the picture. Breathe normally. Relax your body. Hold initially for 5 minutes. Increase the time as you progress in your practice.

OSTEOPOROSIS

Osteoporosis is a condition that occurs when calcium is leached from the bones, causing them to become porous and brittle. Bones and muscles could become damaged as everyday weight-bearing activities become increasingly difficult.

Symptoms of osteoporosis occur most frequently in midlife and, for women, after menopause. People often report lower back pain and muscle spasms. As this disease progresses, the spine can become deformed, causing loss of height. Bones can break quite easily. It is not advisable to jump or engage in any extreme movement because the impact shocks the knee and hip joints.

Osteoporosis can be prevented and treated through regular weight-bearing exercise combined with proper diet and lifestyle. Weight-bearing exercise includes any that require your muscles to work directly against gravity. Meridian exercise is an excellent weight-bearing activity, as it stimulates bone building for the upper and lower body while being a low-impact activity. Start slowly with easier exercises and gradually build up the length of practice time and difficulty of the postures.

SIT-UP (P. 106)

TIPS Perform this exercise slowly, and focus on the movement of your body.

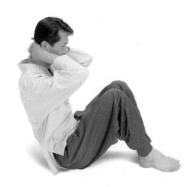

ARM SWINGS (P. 53)

BENEFITS When you swing your arms back and forth, it stimulates and strengthens the muscles and the bones.

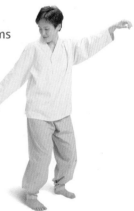

STRADDLE WITH FORWARD BEND AND HIP LIFT (P. 51)

BENEFITS Aligns pelvis and strengthens organs and bones.

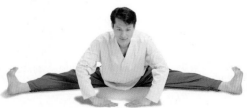

1. STANDING BODY VIBRATION

BENEFITS Prevents and alleviates the symptoms of osteoporosis by enhancing Ki energy and blood circulation to nourish the bone marrow. It also strengthens bones and blood vessels.

1 Stand with your legs shoulder width apart. Place your hands in front of you at waist level with your palms facing each other.

2 Relax your whole body. Keep your fingers straight. Begin to shake your hands and arms. Imagine the vibration coursing through your entire body and notice your body beginning to vibrate as well.

3 Imagine the vibration flowing through the depth of every single cell, from the top of your head down to your toes, nourishing, revitalizing, energizing, and healing you. Vibrate for 5 minutes to start and increase the time with practice.

2. PUSH-UP

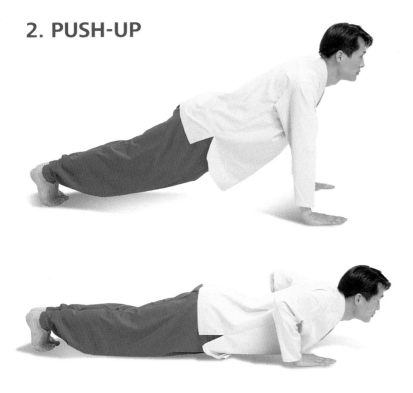

1 Place your palms on the floor and extend your legs behind you, supporting your weight on your arms. Keep your spine elongated and relaxed, and point your toes forward.

2 Bend your arms and descend your chest toward the floor, holding your chest several inches off the floor and focusing on your spine. Hold as long as you can. Increase the time with practice.

SKIN DISORDERS

Scabs, liver spots, and other skin maladies can arise from toxins lodged in the intestines. When the intestines are functioning smoothly, toxins can be eradicated, resulting in radiant and healthy skin. When you perform the recommended intestine exercise and massage your face, ears, and head, oxygenated blood and Ki energy circulation will nourish the tissues, nerves, and cells of the skin.

When your lower extremities are raised, such that your legs are higher than your head, blood flow is expedited to the head and face. The toxins that have accumulated in the liver and kidneys can be released from the body.

Through balancing hormones and boosting oxygen-rich blood flow, meridian exercises give your skin a healthy glow. They keep your skin resilient and prevent dryness. Further, these exercises tone the muscles of your face and neck, preventing excessive sagging.

② Inhale. Slowly raise your right hand to head level and above your head, and push up toward the sky, keeping your palm up all the way. Follow your hand with your eyes.

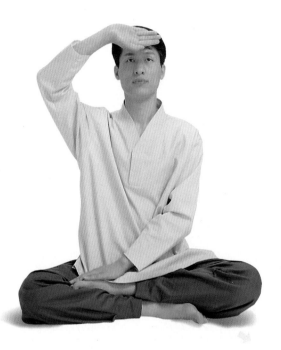

HEADSTAND (P. 34)

TIPS Beginners can try this posture against a wall for more support. As you progress, you may want to attempt this without using the wall. Begin by holding this stance for 20 seconds. Progress to hold the posture 2 minutes with practice. If you have hypertension, heart disease, or glaucoma, it is recommended that you avoid this posture.

1. PUSHING UP THE SKY

BENEFITS This exercise reduces heat energy to the neck and face. It helps pneumonia, bronchitis, palpitations, and other upper respiratory disorders.

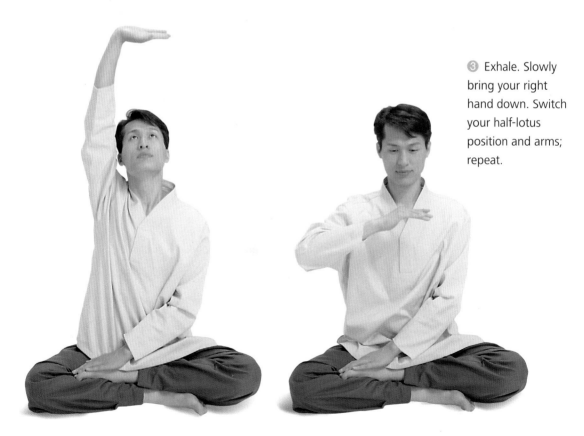

❶ Sit in a half-lotus position, with your left hand covering the left sole of your foot and your right hand placed at your lower abdomen, palm face up.

❸ Exhale. Slowly bring your right hand down. Switch your half-lotus position and arms; repeat.

2. LYING LEG ROTATION

❶ Prior to beginning this exercise, perform the neck exercise to increase the flexibility in your neck. Then place a soft mat or cushion on the floor and gently rest the top of your head on it. Extend your legs behind you with the toes pointing forward, and place your palms on the floor at chest height and at a 45–degree angle from your body.

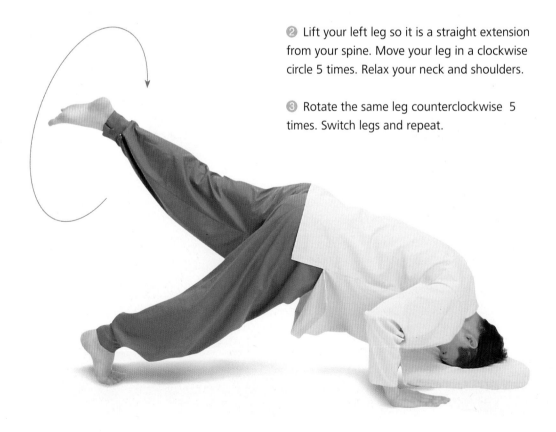

❷ Lift your left leg so it is a straight extension from your spine. Move your leg in a clockwise circle 5 times. Relax your neck and shoulders.

❸ Rotate the same leg counterclockwise 5 times. Switch legs and repeat.

3. SWEEPING THE FACE

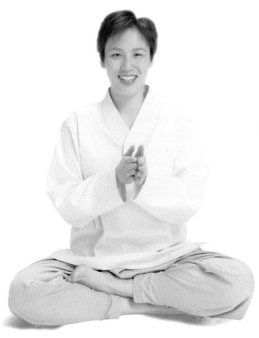

① Sit in a half-lotus position. Take 3 deep breaths. Inhale. Rub your hands until you feel heat energy.

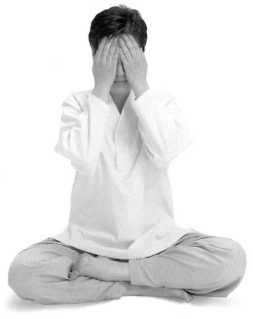

② Exhale and sweep your face. Start at your forehead and sweep in a downward motion, including the ears, cheeks, and bridge of the nose. Imagine you are washing your face. It is best to perform this about 5 minutes before you go to sleep.

4. BICYCLE EXERCISE

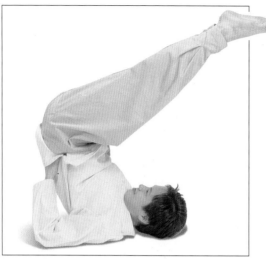

SKIN DISORDERS

❷ Support your waist with both hands. Straighten your legs so they are perpendicular to the floor, keeping your knees soft.

❶ Lie on your back. Raise both of your legs straight above your hips, and use your hands to raise your trunk as well.

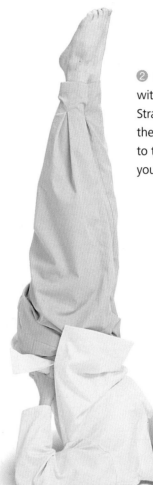

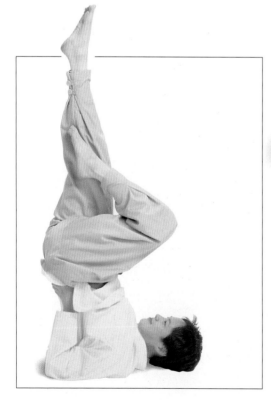

❸ Begin to move your legs as if you are riding a bicycle, moving at a comfortable and gentle pace. Relax your neck and your shoulders. Continue riding for as long as possible, but up to 5 minutes.

5. SCALP ENERGIZER

TIPS Perform this exercise on the floor or on a hard bed. You will achieve more beneficial results from this exercise the longer you are able to maintain the bending position. This exercise appears very simple, but it is challenging to execute. It is important to progress gently, comfortably, and at your own pace. As you continue to practice, you will notice you can extend your bending time as well as your reach.

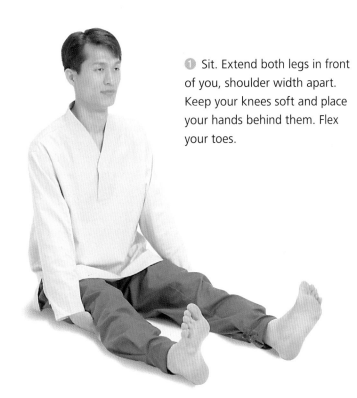

❶ Sit. Extend both legs in front of you, shoulder width apart. Keep your knees soft and place your hands behind them. Flex your toes.

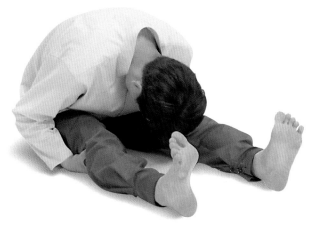

❷ Inhale. Bend forward from your hips, moving your torso toward your legs. Bend as far as is comfortable and hold for as long as you can.

❸ Exhale and sit up. Repeat the movement 10 times.

6. EXERCISE TO REDUCE ITCHING

BENEFITS Helps blood and Ki energy circulation in the shoulders and back. Releases pain from the neck, shoulders, and arms, and relieves discomfort in the ears. Also alleviates itchiness.

TIPS It is important to extend your arms and to pull them back as much as possible to open the chest. Keep your spine extended but not rigid.

SKIN DISORDERS

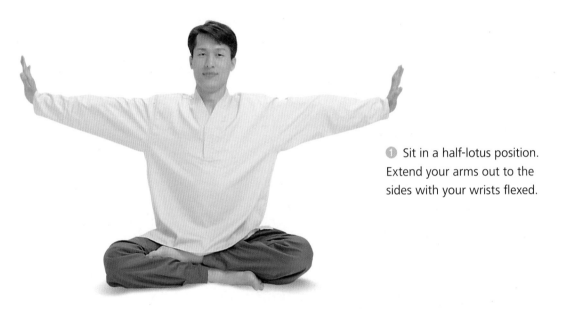

❶ Sit in a half-lotus position. Extend your arms out to the sides with your wrists flexed.

❷ Inhale. Keeping your arms extended, bring them to the center with your palms facing outward. Turn your head to the side, very slowly, as far as possible. Follow the movement with your eyes.

❸ Exhale. Turn your head to the center and then to the opposite direction. Repeat the exercise 20 times.

❹ When you complete this exercise, perform the backward neck tilt (page 67) 36 times. While swallowing your saliva, focus on your lower abdomen.

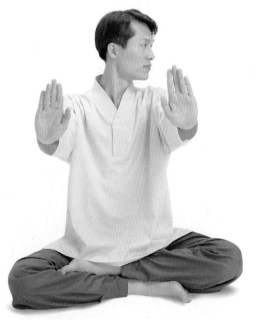

7. FACIAL REJUVENATION

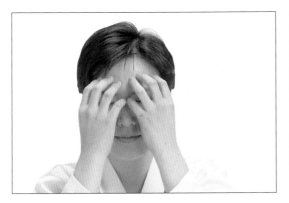 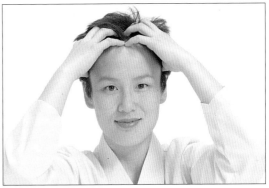

① Sit on the floor and place your fingertips on your forehead. Gently perform a raking and massaging movement down toward your eyebrows.

② Repeat this in the opposite direction, moving from your eyebrows upward and over your scalp.

8. NOSE MASSAGE

TIP This exercise is best done before going to sleep because it can cause redness around the nose.

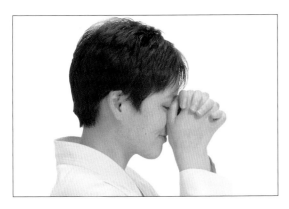 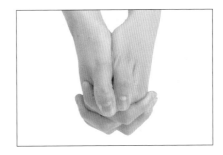

Lock your fingers and place the pads of your hands around your nose. Pull forward on the cartilage of the nose and hold for 2 minutes. You will notice the effects of this exercise after about one or two months if you practice daily.

9. UPPER BODY LIFT AND LEG ROTATION

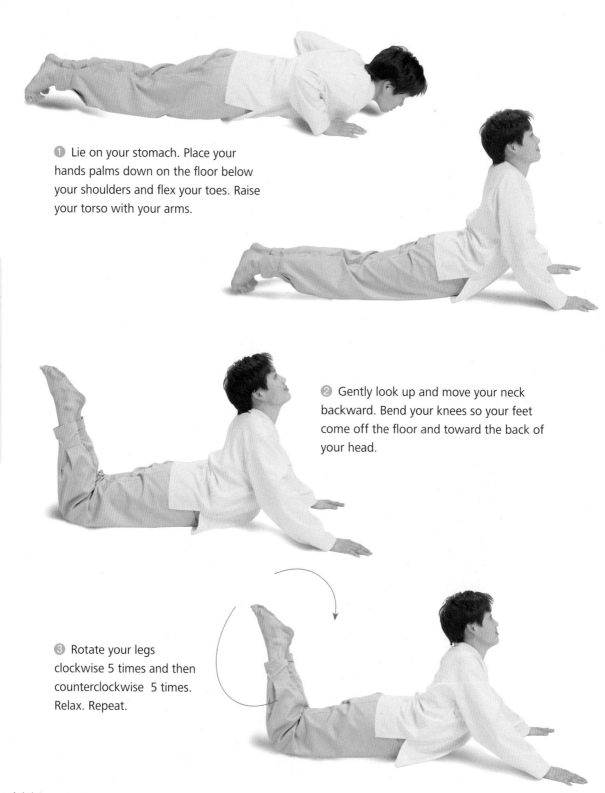

1 Lie on your stomach. Place your hands palms down on the floor below your shoulders and flex your toes. Raise your torso with your arms.

2 Gently look up and move your neck backward. Bend your knees so your feet come off the floor and toward the back of your head.

3 Rotate your legs clockwise 5 times and then counterclockwise 5 times. Relax. Repeat.

10. SMOOTHING EYE WRINKLES

BENEFITS Supplies moisture to the skin around the eyes by enhancing the blood and Ki energy circulation to this area.

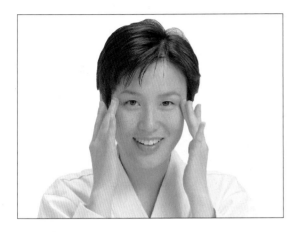

Place your middle finger on your temples. Massage in a clockwise motion until the area feels moist.

11. BREATHING TECHNIQUE

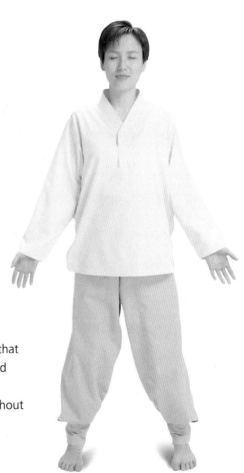

❶ You can perform this exercise while standing or lying down. If you are standing, bend your knees 15 degrees. If you are lying down, stand with your feet shoulder width apart and your arms to your sides, about 30 degrees from your body, palms facing forward. Close your eyes and relax your whole body.

❷ Breathe softly and gently. Focus on your mind.

❸ When you exhale through your mouth, imagine that your skin pores open and stagnant energy is released through them. When you inhale through your nose, imagine allowing fresh Ki energy to circulate throughout your body, from head to toes.

BONE, MUSCLE, AND SKIN

HAIR LOSS

Under normal circumstances, people lose an average of seventy to eighty hairs daily. Hair loss greater than this could indicate alopecia. When experiencing alopecia, hair loss can result from pulling on your hair, braiding it, or brushing it roughly. Hair loss is often noticed between six weeks and three months following a high fever. Medications for thyroid disorders, heart disease, cancer, and arthritis may result in hair loss as well. In addition, hair loss may occur two to three months following major surgical intervention, as well as postpartum. Stress and emotional disorders also exacerbate the probability of hair loss.

Eastern Medicine practitioners believe that hair loss is related to kidney dysfunction. If you have normal or active kidney function, which is accompanied by heightened stamina, this will be reflected in healthy hair.

Practicing abdominal breathing inhibits accelerated aging, promoting a healthy scalp and better hair growth. It is recommended that you supplement the exercises in this section with exercises that promote healthy kidney functioning.

SITTING FORWARD BEND (P. 50)

BENEFITS Strengthens kidney functioning and treats alopecia, which promotes growth of healthy hair.

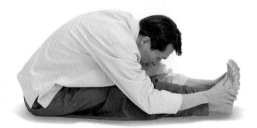

1. LYING KNEE BEND

① Kneel with the buttocks on your heels and your toes pointing behind you. Place your palms facedown on your knees.

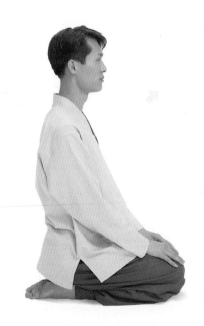

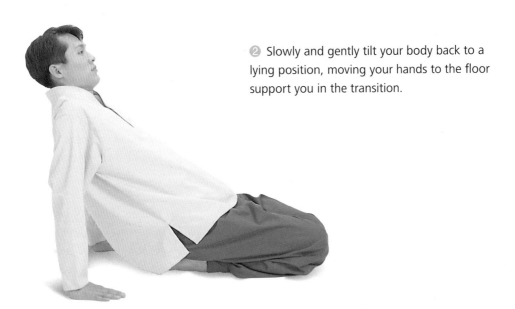

❷ Slowly and gently tilt your body back to a lying position, moving your hands to the floor support you in the transition.

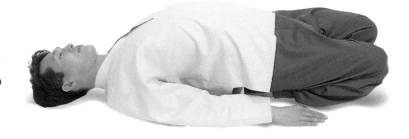

❸ While lying back on the floor, tilt your head back and touch the top of your head to the floor. Raise your chest and waist. Hold for a few seconds.

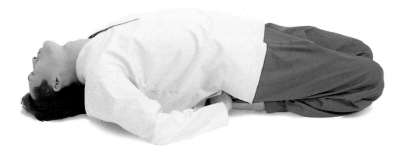

❹ Slowly release. Repeat several times, as comfortable.

Bone, Muscle, and Skin   *147*

2. SCALP STIMULATION

BENEFITS Strengthens hair roots and results in better hair luster.

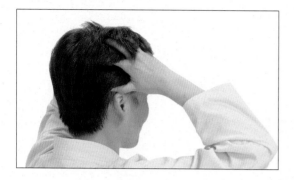

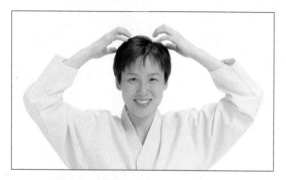

❶ Using your fingertips, gently tap the circumference of the head. If you have damaged or brittle hair, or if your hair breaks easily, tap very lightly.

❷ Gently rake your fingers through your hair, beginning at the hairline around the ears. Move up toward the top of your head and over to the back. Gently move from the hairline at the top of your forehead to the top of the head and then to the back of the head. Also, move to the hairline at the back of the neck and rake up toward the top of the head. Focus on your scalp and the calming of your mind.

3. CURLING INTO A BALL

❶ Sit with your feet flat on the floor and your knees in front of your chest. Embrace your knees with both of your arms. Inhale. Focus on your lower abdomen. Gently pull your knees toward your chest while simultaneously bending from your hips to enable your chest to meet your knees. Lower your head gently to touch your face to your knees.

❷ Hold for a few seconds. Relax your body. Exhale and release. Repeat as often as you are comfortable.

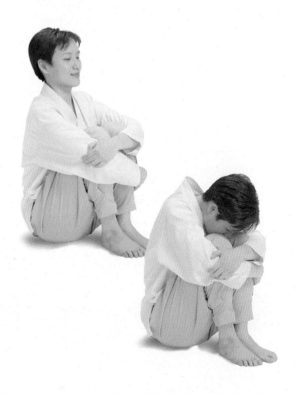

4. EXERCISE FOR HAIR GROWTH

BENEFITS Promotes blood and Ki energy circulation to the head while strengthening the kidneys.

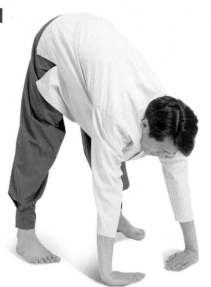

❶ Stand with your feet slightly wider than shoulder width apart. Bend from the hips and place your palms on the floor, fingers pointing toward each other, about a foot in front of your toes. Keep your knees soft. Gently bounce 8 times.

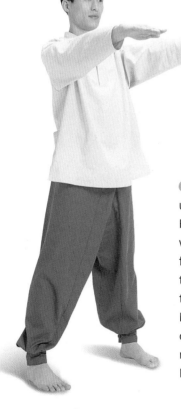

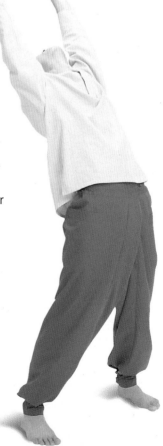

❷ Slowly and gently raise your upper body to standing. Inhale. Raise your arms in front of you with your palms facing the floor first. Sweep them overhead so they face the sky as you gently tilt your upper body backward. Hold for a few seconds. Focus on your kidneys. Exhale and return to position in STEP 1. Repeat 5 times very slowly.

PULLING KNEE TOWARD THE CHEST (P. 87)

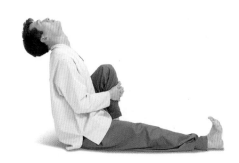

HEART DISEASE

Heart disease, also known as cardiovascular disease, includes a number of conditions affecting the heart: congestive heart failure, congenital heart disease, and heart attack, among others. Heart disease is the leading cause of death in the United States.

Eastern Medicine proposes that when there is an imbalance of Ki energy circulation near the heart, it is accompanied by a sense of sadness, while a balance of Ki energy in the heart promotes a sense of joy. Those afflicted with heart disease tend to exhibit irritable, rigid, and compulsive behaviors. Emotions become unstable and can result in a constriction of the arterial flow, high blood pressure, and heart palpitations. Keys to preventing heart disease include quitting smoking, improving cholesterol, controlling high blood pressure, maintaining a healthy weight, and exercising.

If you have been diagnosed with heart disease, breathe in the opposite fashion to that which is normally described for the meridian exercises. Because most postures instruct you to inhale as you begin a motion, if you have heart disease, you should exhale as you begin the motion and inhale to return to the original posture.

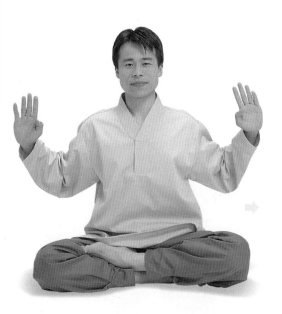

② Inhale. Keep your elbows bent as you open your hands and bring your arms out to the side as far as is comfortable. Focus on opening your chest.

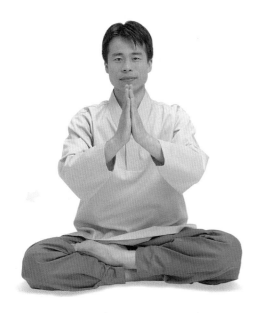

1. EXPANDING THE CHEST

BENEFITS Promotes deep and full breathing and enhances heart and lung capacity. If you sit and hold the positions in STEPs 2 and 4 for 10 minutes or more, this can help to realign the spine and bones. Keep your spine straightened and focus on your heart. Ki and blood circulation will be strengthened, as will your heart.

TIP If you experience palpitations or difficulty breathing, perform the movements and just breathe naturally and comfortably.

① Sit in a half-lotus position. Place both hands in the prayer position in front of your chest.

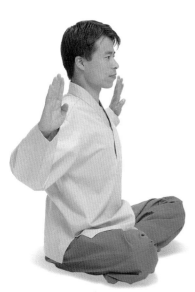

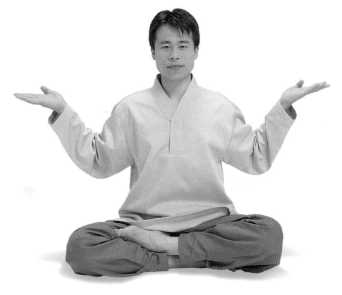

③ Keep your spine lengthened while holding your breath. Gently pull your shoulder blades toward each other and hold for 10 seconds.

④ Exhale and bring your hands together in the prayer position, as in STEP 1. Inhale and slowly pull your arms apart again as far as you comfortably can, this time with your wrists flexed and palms face up. Remember to keep your spine lengthened and your neck and shoulders relaxed. Focus on your heart. Repeat several times.

2. HALF-LOTUS FORWARD BEND

BENEFITS Relieves tightness in chest and promotes deep and full breathing capacity.

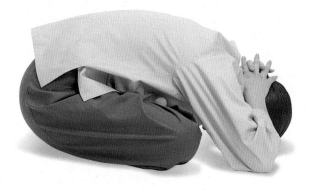

❶ Sit in a half-lotus position. Interlace your fingers behind your neck. Inhale. Bend your upper body forward and touch the floor with your forehead and elbows.

HEART DISEASE

❷ Hold this position for as long as you comfortably can. Exhale, sit up, and expand your chest as you return to the original posture.

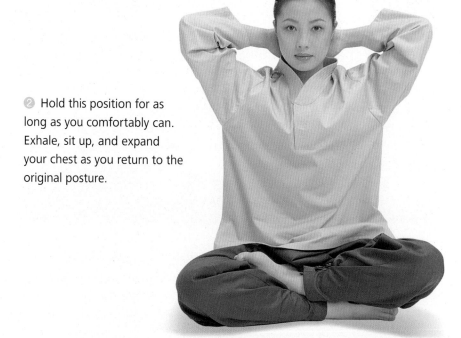

3. SITTING SIDE BEND

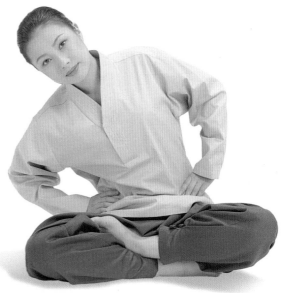

① Sit in a half-lotus position with your hands on each side of your waist. Inhale. Slowly and gently bend to the left. Hold for a few seconds.

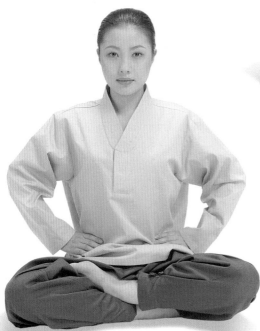

② Exhale. Inhale and bend to the right. Hold for a few seconds. Exhale to the original posture.

③ Repeat 5 times.

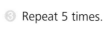

4. ARM TWIST

BENEFITS Helps to release stiffness in the arms and shoulders associated with heart difficulty. Activates the Pericardium Meridian (see page 332, #9) and the Heart Meridian (see page 330, #5).

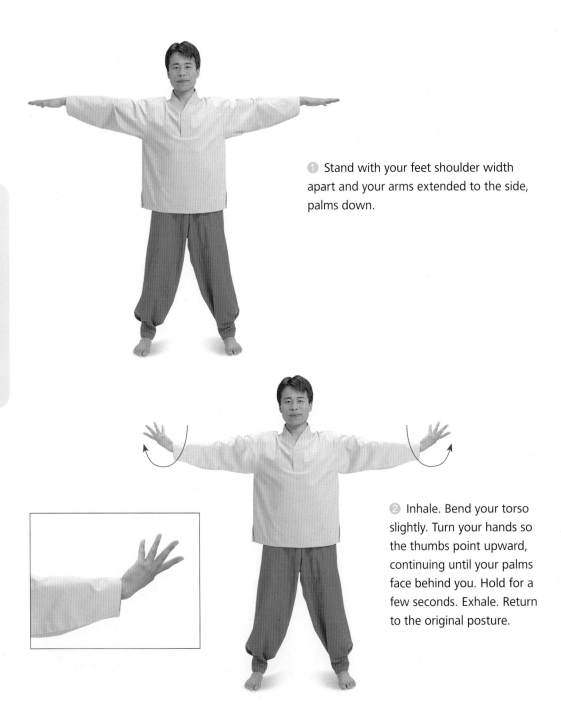

① Stand with your feet shoulder width apart and your arms extended to the side, palms down.

② Inhale. Bend your torso slightly. Turn your hands so the thumbs point upward, continuing until your palms face behind you. Hold for a few seconds. Exhale. Return to the original posture.

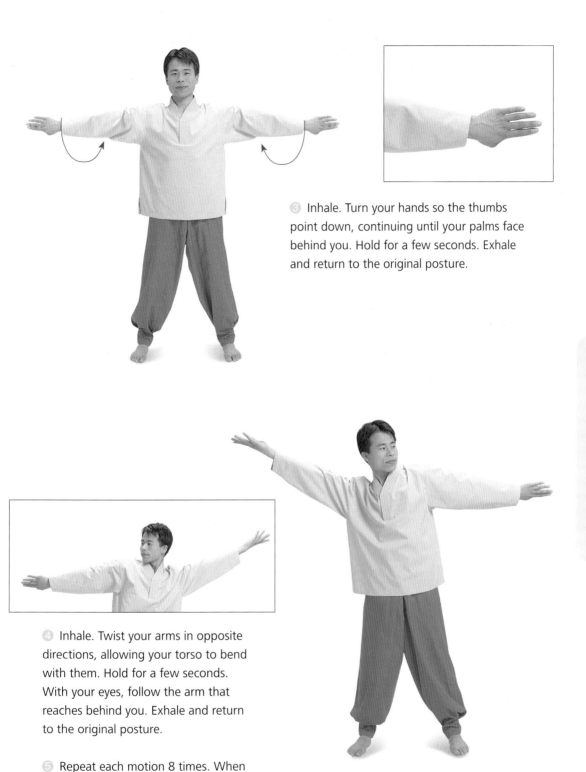

③ Inhale. Turn your hands so the thumbs point down, continuing until your palms face behind you. Hold for a few seconds. Exhale and return to the original posture.

④ Inhale. Twist your arms in opposite directions, allowing your torso to bend with them. Hold for a few seconds. With your eyes, follow the arm that reaches behind you. Exhale and return to the original posture.

⑤ Repeat each motion 8 times. When you finish, massage your muscles from your shoulders to your wrists.

5. PRESSING THE SOLE

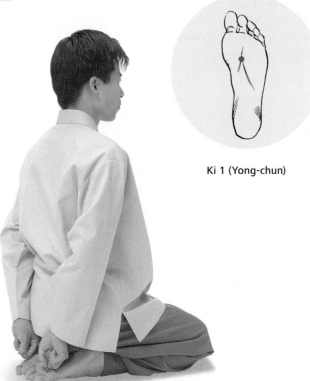

Ki 1 (Yong-chun)

① Kneel with your buttocks on your heels and your knees comfortably separated. Make fists with both of your hands and use the middle joint of the third finger to press the Ki 1 acupressure point on your sole.

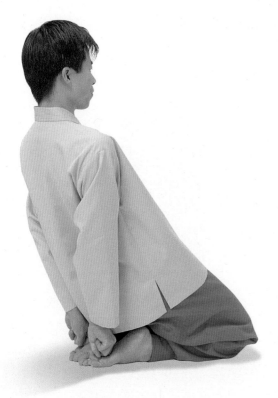

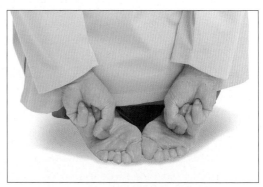

② Inhale. Lean backward with your weight on your hands as you gently lift your hips, pressing the Ki 1 acupressure point. Hold for about 7 seconds. Exhale. Repeat 5 times.

6. ARCHER EXERCISE

TIPS Keep your upper torso facing straight ahead. Follow the movements with your eyes and head. Relax the neck and shoulders.

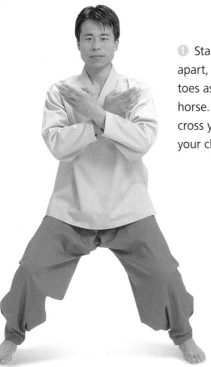

① Stand with your feet wide apart, knees bent over your toes as if you were riding a horse. Bend your elbows and cross your forearms in front of your chest.

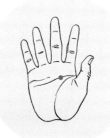

PC 8 (Jang-shim)

② Inhale. Extend your left arm to the left side and flex your wrist. Follow the movement with your eyes and head. Bend your right elbow while making a fist with your right hand. Gently glide the right arm, like an archer, as far back as is comfortable, while you feel your chest expand. Continue to inhale. Imagine Ki energy flowing into the PC 8 acupressure point through the arm and chest and down to the lower abdomen.

③ Exhale. Return to the original posture and repeat with your other arm. Do 5 sets with each arm.

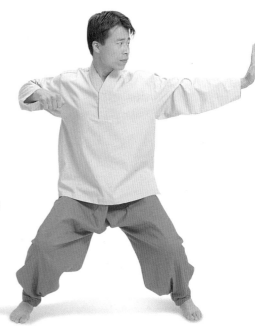

7. WHOLE BODY RELAXATION

BENEFITS Promotes relaxation of the body and mind while enhancing blood circulation. Facilitates alpha brain wave function, assisting in self-healing for hypertension, insomnia, and other autonomic nervous system disorders.

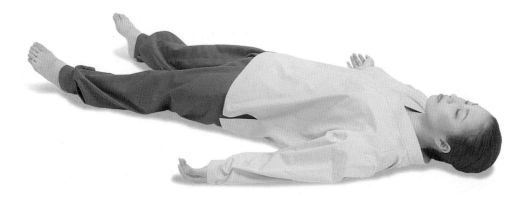

❶ Lie on your back. Place your feet shoulder width apart and your arms at a 45-degree angle, palms facing up. Close your eyes.

❷ With your mind's eye, scan your face, neck, shoulders, arms, hands, fingers, chest, lower abdomen, back, hips, legs, feet, and toes, and note where you experience tension.

❸ Imagine the bright light of the sun melting the icy streams of winter as you begin to see the waters flowing with the guiding light of the sun. Focus your mind upon releasing any tension you may experience in your body.

❹ Imagine now that your body is warmer and that your head is cooler than the rest of your body. Breathe naturally and comfortably throughout this exercise. As you become more relaxed, your breathing will become slower and deeper.

8. BREATHING FOR THE HEART

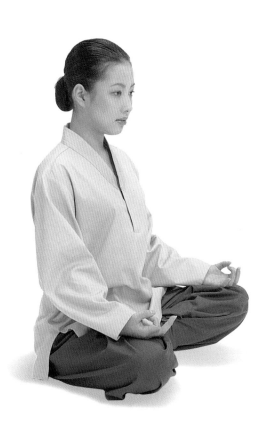

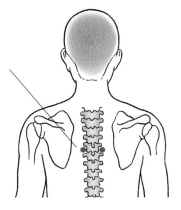

BL 15 (Shim-yu)

The BL 15 acupressure points are located along the left and right sides of the fifth vertebra of the thoracic spine. There is about a 2-inch space between the two acupressure points. The Heart Meridian flows through these two points to the brain. If there is a blockage, they can become inflamed and cause heart disease.

① Sit in a half-lotus position with the backs of your hands resting on your knees and your thumbs and index fingertips touching, as shown in the picture. Focus on the Bl 15 acupressure points and the heart, imagining the Ki energy flow connecting the heart and Bl 15 points as you breathe slowly and gently. Hold the pose for 15-20 minutes. As you breathe, experience your chest accumulating Ki energy and your heart becoming stronger.

9. HOLDING UP HEAVEN

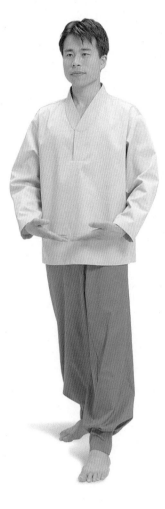

❶ Stand with your left foot straight in front of you and your right foot at a 45-degree angle. Place your hands near your lower abdomen, palms facing up and fingertips pointing toward one another.

❷ Inhale. Gently lift your arms, keeping your palms facing up. When your hands reach chin level, rotate your hands so the fingertips point away from you, and then rotate them around to your shoulders, still raising your hands. When your hands move above your head, point your fingertips toward one another again, extending your arms completely. Follow the motion with your eyes, gazing at the backs of your hands.

❸ Exhale. Bring your hands down to the original posture. Switch the position of your feet and repeat the exercise.

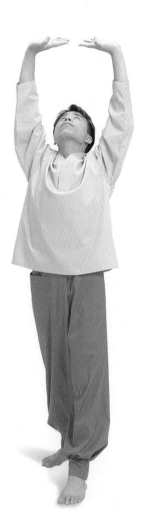

10. SOLE CLAPPING

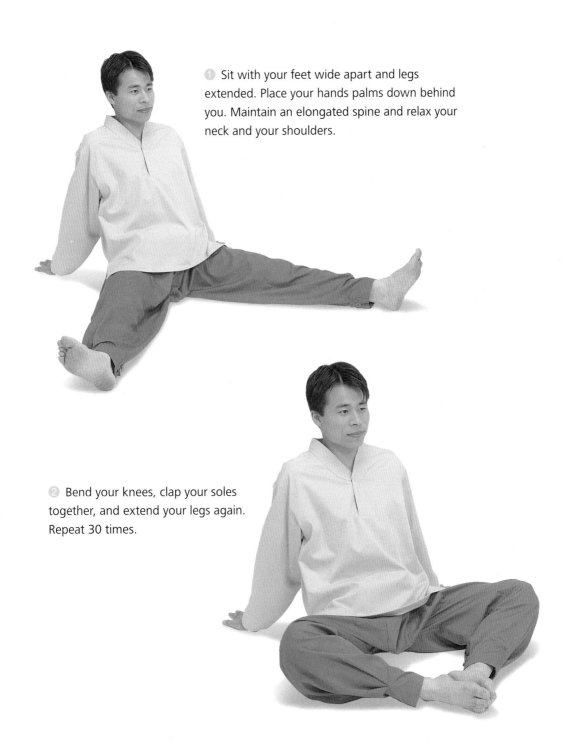

① Sit with your feet wide apart and legs extended. Place your hands palms down behind you. Maintain an elongated spine and relax your neck and your shoulders.

② Bend your knees, clap your soles together, and extend your legs again. Repeat 30 times.

11. WAIST LIFTING

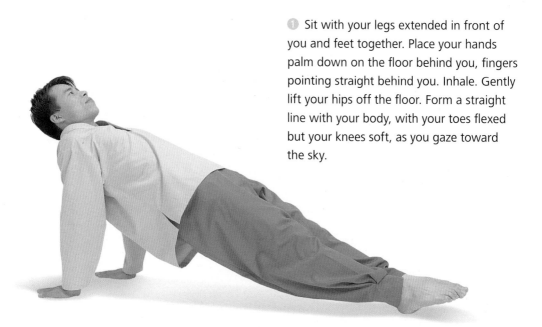

① Sit with your legs extended in front of you and feet together. Place your hands palm down on the floor behind you, fingers pointing straight behind you. Inhale. Gently lift your hips off the floor. Form a straight line with your body, with your toes flexed but your knees soft, as you gaze toward the sky.

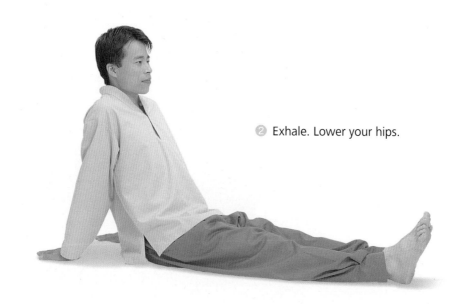

② Exhale. Lower your hips.

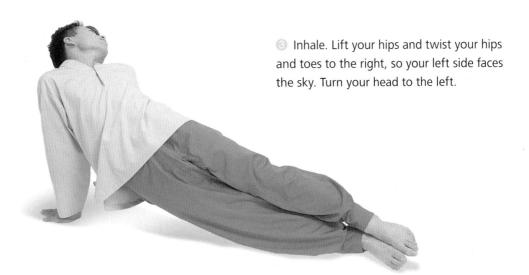

3 Inhale. Lift your hips and twist your hips and toes to the right, so your left side faces the sky. Turn your head to the left.

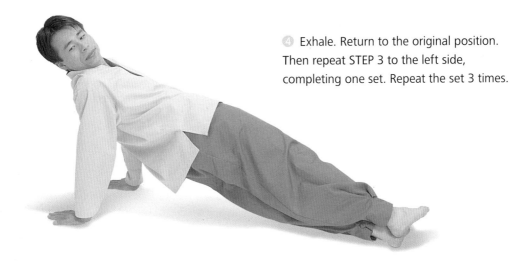

4 Exhale. Return to the original position. Then repeat STEP 3 to the left side, completing one set. Repeat the set 3 times.

HIGH BLOOD PRESSURE

Hypertension is often referred to as high blood pressure, and symptoms include headaches, anxiety, ringing in the ears, shortness of breath, tightness in the chest, tingling or numbness in the legs, nose bleeds, and a sensation of pressure at the back of the neck.

A hallmark in the self-healing treatment for hypertension is the ability to mitigate tension and anxiety through relaxation, meditation, and the meridian exercises recommended in this chapter. Through this practice, blood vessels, which are constricted when afflicted with hypertension, can begin to relax. Breathing and meditation exercises are best accomplished in a lying down position.

When performing meridian exercises, breathe naturally. Headstands are not recommended because blood can rush to the brain quickly and exacerbate the hypertension. As you progress in the meridian exercises, you will experience increased warmth in the body as the blood vessels lessen their constriction and begin to open.

WHOLE BODY TAPPING (P. 20)

BENEFITS Releases stagnant energy throughout the body. Enhances blood and Ki energy circulation.

TIPS Beginners are cautioned to pat gently and comfortably. As you progress, the patting can be applied with more pressure.

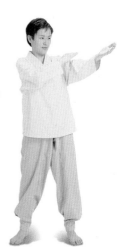

CIRCULATION EXERCISE (P. 24)

BENEFITS Releases stagnant energy that has accumulated in the body. Enhances peripheral circulation of blood to the heart, thereby lowering blood pressure.

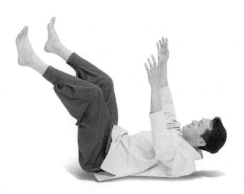

1. STIMULATING PALMS AND SOLES

BENEFITS Enhances blood and Ki energy circulation because the palms of the hands and the soles of the feet are connected to the respiratory and circulatory system and their adjacent organs. Helpful in relieving the symptoms of hypertension or hypotension as well as for clearing the mind.

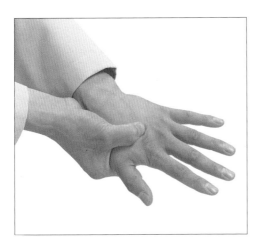

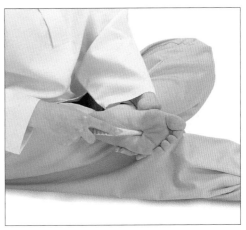

① When you stimulate your palms, first locate the PC 8 (Jang-shim) acupressure points in your palms, below the lowest finger joint and between the index and middle finger metatarsals. Then turn your hand and touch the spot opposite the PC 8. Press with your thumb as shown in the picture and begin to massage firmly.

② When you stimulate the soles of your feet, bring one ankle across the opposite knee, so you can reach the sole. Make a fist with your hand and pat or hit the sole of your foot. Locate the Ki 1 (Yong-chun) acupressure points below the ball of your foot and between the first two metatarsals and press with your thumb. You can also use a wooden acupressure point stick. Massage and press these points for at least 10 minutes per day for optimal results.

2. PALM AND SOLE BREATHING

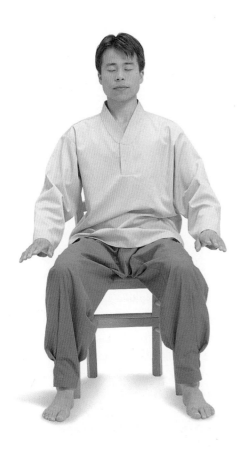

❶ Sit in a chair with your spine straight and your neck and shoulders relaxed. Place your feet flat on the floor, and bend your arms at your sides with your palms down, as if your palms were resting on the arms of the chair.

❷ Close your eyes. Focus on the centers of the palms and centers of the soles as you breathe. Imagine a continuous flow of Ki energy through these points.

❸ Continue to breathe like this for 15-20 minutes. Notice the relaxation spread throughout your body.

3. DEEP RELAXATION BREATHING

BENEFITS Enhances Ki energy and blood circulation. Boosts immune function, thereby expediting the self-healing process. Through mindful focus, you can become aware of the sensation of the Ki energy flowing throughout your body.

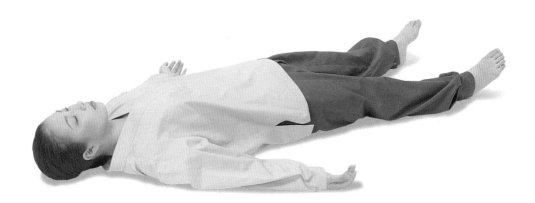

❶ Lie on your back comfortably with your feet shoulder width apart and your hands relaxed at your sides. Scan your body with your mind's eye, imagining it as a block of ice with the warm sun radiating upon it. Imagine the warm rays of the sun melting the ice, first at the top of your head, then on your forehead, face, throat, neck, chest, back, hip joints, buttocks, backs and fronts of your thighs, legs, feet, toes, shoulders, arms, hands, and fingers. Imagine your body becoming a flowing stream of water. Scan your body for any part that needs further melting and focus on it until you experience it transforming into flowing water.

❷ Relax your whole body. Begin to become increasingly more relaxed and comfortable. Notice your breath becoming deeper and slower. Focus on your heart. Feel the warmth. Repeat to yourself three times, "My mind is becoming more and more comfortable."

❸ Imagine warm energy flowing through your Conception Vessel to your lower abdomen. Continue breathing comfortably, becoming more and more relaxed.

4. ACUPRESSURE FOR HYPERTENSION

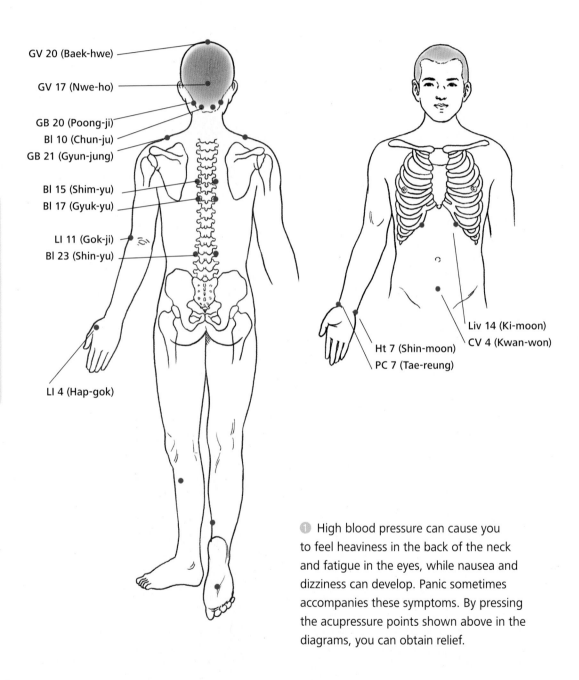

GV 20 (Baek-hwe)
GV 17 (Nwe-ho)
GB 20 (Poong-ji)
Bl 10 (Chun-ju)
GB 21 (Gyun-jung)
Bl 15 (Shim-yu)
Bl 17 (Gyuk-yu)
LI 11 (Gok-ji)
Bl 23 (Shin-yu)
LI 4 (Hap-gok)

Liv 14 (Ki-moon)
CV 4 (Kwan-won)
Ht 7 (Shin-moon)
PC 7 (Tae-reung)

❶ High blood pressure can cause you to feel heaviness in the back of the neck and fatigue in the eyes, while nausea and dizziness can develop. Panic sometimes accompanies these symptoms. By pressing the acupressure points shown above in the diagrams, you can obtain relief.

5. STRENGTHENING THE HEART MERIDIAN

BENEFITS Stimulates the Heart Meridian as it strengthens the small and large intestines.

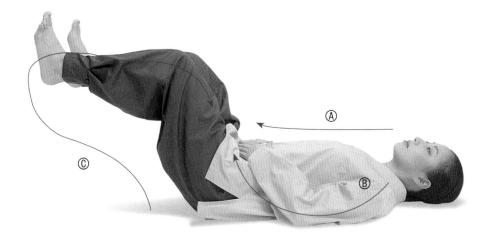

① Lie on your back with your legs extended. Raise your knees above your hips and flex your ankles to 90 degrees. Relax your neck and shoulders. Place both hands on your lower abdomen with your thumbs and index fingers touching to form a triangle.

② Breathe gently and use your mind's eye to scan your body in the following progression:
A: face, neck, chest, upper abdomen
B: shoulders, arms, lower abdomen
C: both thighs, legs, toes, soles, knees, and thighs

③ Focus on your lower abdomen. Perform abdominal breathing. When you inhale, focus on the energy coming through the center of the sole to your lower abdomen. When you exhale, focus on the stagnant energy from the lower abdomen releasing through the toes. If concentrating is difficult for you at this time, go back to STEP 3 and practice by focusing with your mind's eye. Return to abdominal breathing.

HYPOTENSION
(Low Blood Pressure)

The conditions of hypotension and hypertension are both related to the malfunctioning of the blood vessels. Symptoms of hypotension include chronic fatigue, dizziness, difficulty with memory and concentration, heart palpitations, tightness or pain in the chest, pale face, weak and slow pulse, and coldness in the hands and feet. Eventually the body functions can be compromised as a result of continued hypotension. Also, when you arise suddenly from a sitting position, you may experience dizziness and, in the extreme case, you may lose consciousness. When you awake from sleep, you could experience decreased motivation to participate in life's activities.

The meridian exercises recommended in this chapter, combined with breathing exercises, will help to ease the symptoms of hypotension by enhancing the heart's ability to circulate oxygenated blood to the organs and extremities. As you progress gradually through these exercises, increase practice and posture time.

SHOULDERSTAND WITH WAIST SUPPORT (P. 70)

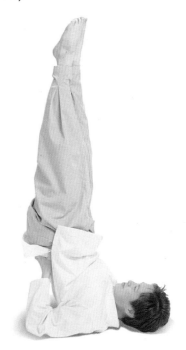

UPPER BODY LIFT (P. 105)

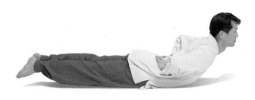

PUSH-UP (P. 135)

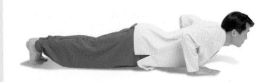

1. WHEELBARROW POSTURE

TIPS Avoid this exercise if you have hypertension or heart disease.

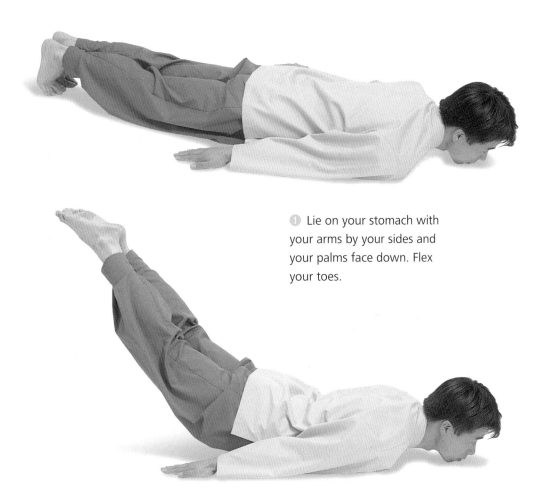

❶ Lie on your stomach with your arms by your sides and your palms face down. Flex your toes.

❷ Inhale. As you hold your breath, flex your lower abdomen. Push with your hands while lifting both of your legs in the air as high as is comfortable for your lower back. Use your lower abdomen and hands to support you.

❸ Hold this position for several seconds or for as long as you can, and exhale slowly while bringing your legs down gently. Repeat 3 the movement 3 times.

2. SQUATS

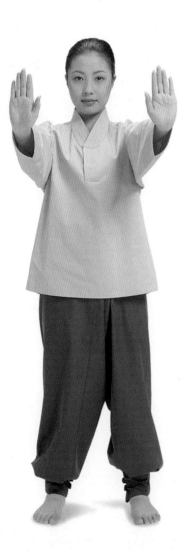

① Stand with your feet shoulder width apart and your spine straightened. Relax your neck and shoulders. Extend both arms forward at shoulder level with both of your wrists flexed.

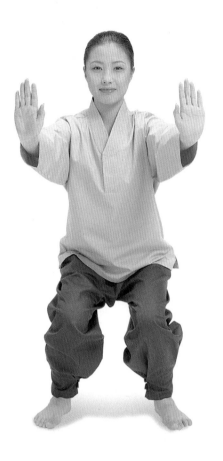

② Bend your knees and lower your body as if preparing to sit. Rise slowly to STEP 1 position. Repeat 20 times.

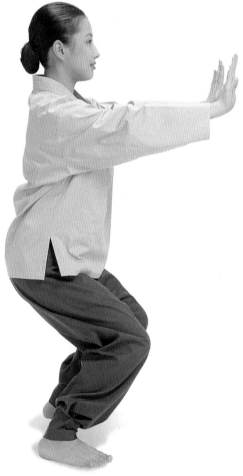

③ Keep your spine straight and, while you are bending as if to sit, keep your knees at a 90-degree angle.

STROKE

The human brain houses an intricate vascular webbing and a communication system for the well-being of the rest of the body, and it operates on a continuous flow of oxygen and nutrients from the blood. If the blood flow becomes restricted or clotted, brain tissue can die from the lack of oxygen. This is called an ischemic stroke and is the most common kind of stroke. A hemorrhagic stroke, also known as an aneurysm, occurs when the cerebral artery ruptures. A transient ischemic attack (TIA) is a more benign form of stroke but can be a warning sign of health problems that could lead to a more severe form of stroke.

The onset of a stroke is usually signaled by numbness in the hands and feet, weakness in facial muscles on one side, insomnia, dizziness, shortness of breath, sudden severe headache, difficulty with visual acuity, difficulty maintaining coordination and balance, and dysarthria—difficulty articulating due to muscle damage to the peripheral or central nervous system.

Stroke can leave lasting effects, including paralysis or weakness, dysarthria and other language problems, poststroke depression, pain, and learning and memory deficiencies. It is imperative that preventive measures be taken based on current medical knowledge regarding health care in order to reduce the possibility of a stroke. Pay careful attention to the warning signs of stroke, including high blood pressure, diabetes, high cholesterol, irregular heartbeat or other heart conditions, and a history of TIAs.

These exercises should be performed with patience if you have experienced a stroke. Keeping your body active is crucial, and long periods of immobility are not recommended. One activity to help circulation is to place two walnuts in your hand while moving and rubbing your hands together, rotating the walnuts. In addition, energy healing and massage are helpful for poststroke rehabilitation to enhance energy and blood circulation.

WHOLE BODY PATTING
(P. 20)

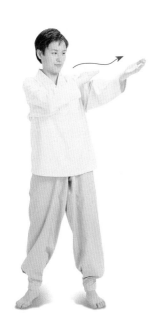

CIRCULATION EXERCISE
(P. 24)

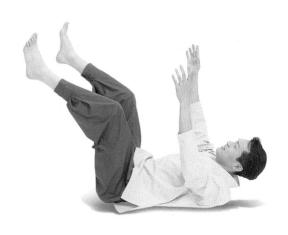

PENDULUM SWING
(P. 45)

TOE TAPPING
(P. 32)

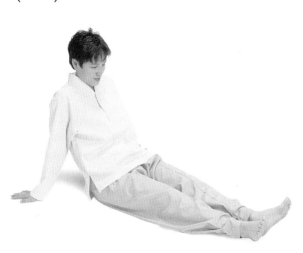

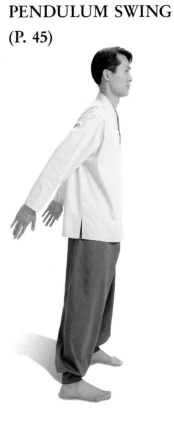

1. HAND RUBBING

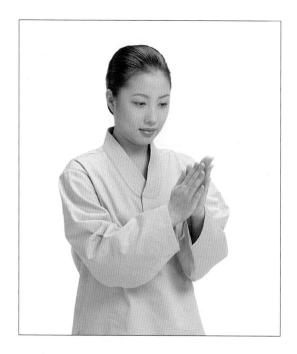

● Cup your hands together so that the Jang-shim acupressure points in the center of the palms do not touch. Rub your hands together quickly to create heat. Count to 10, and then stop for a few seconds before beginning to rub again. Repeat 10 times.

2. FINGER COMB

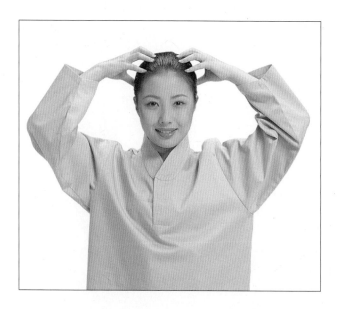

● Relax. Spread your fingers and place the tips on your head. Comb your fingers through your hair, beginning at the forehead and moving toward the back of the head. Then press with your fingers all around your head.

3. SUPERMAN POSTURE

BENEFITS Helps to accumulate and strengthen Ki energy throughout the body while opening the energy blockages and strengthening the autonomic nervous system. Assists in optimal functioning of the organs and enhances circulation, minimizing the chance of stroke.

TIPS Perform this exercise comfortably. Do not force yourself to maintain the posture. With practice you will be able to hold the posture over longer periods of time.

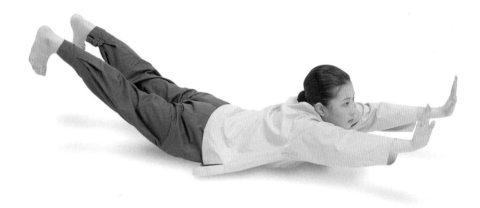

❶ Lie on your stomach with your arms reaching out in front of you.

❷ Inhale. Lift your head up. Looking straight ahead, arch your back, and lift your hands and feet. Tense your wrists and ankles so they make 90-degree angles with your arms and legs. With advanced practice, you can employ abdominal breathing to enhance the benefits of this exercise.

❸ Exhale. Relax your body as you let it return to the floor. Repeat.

❹ This posture is very difficult, particularly in the initial phases of your learning. With practice and concentration, you will be able to balance Ki energy flow. Observe your body condition and perform the posture daily if you can. If you experience shaking, this signals the release of energy blockages. Maintain this posture for 2 minutes or less in the beginning, depending on your body condition. With practice you can increase this to 30 minutes or more.

GASTROINTESTINAL DISORDERS

Gastrointestinal (GI) disorders affect the digestive system, which then affects your overall well-being. Symptoms may include diarrhea, constipation, bleeding from the digestive tract, regurgitation, difficulty swallowing, abdominal pain, flatulence, loss of appetite, and nausea.

Negative emotions and worrisome thoughts are often internalized within the gastrointestinal system, impairing its ability to function properly. Practice abdominal breathing to calm the mind and body, control Ki energy, and minimize the opportunity for emotions to affect your digestion. Try closing your eyes and using your mind's eye to scan your body from the top of your head down to your toes. As you concentrate in this way, you are helping to bring fire energy down to the lower abdomen to aid in digestion.

By performing abdominal breathing, your abdomen will become warm with Ki energy surges. Blockages are released and maximal functioning of the stomach and other vital organs can be achieved. Continuous practice will help you to achieve a balance of Water Up, Fire Down.

LEW TAPPING (P. 36)

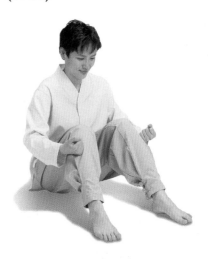

BODY WITH BEND AND TWIST (P. 72)

BENEFITS Eases swelling and bloating, facilitates weight loss, regulates appetite, releases excess fat from abdomen and thighs, helps to control diabetes, and realigns lumbar vertebrae and sacrum.

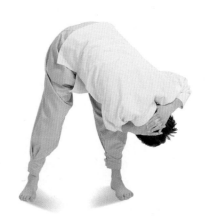

PUSHING UP THE SKY
(P. 137)

BENEFITS Releases stagnant energy from associated energy blocks in the abdomen. Enhances stomach functioning.

TIPS Press one hand on the sole of your foot. As you raise your other hand, follow the back of the hand with your eyes.

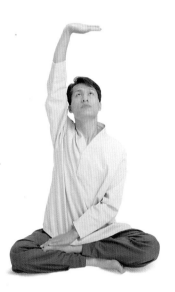

1. ABDOMINAL BREATHING FOR WEAK STOMACH

BENEFITS Accumulates heat energy in the lower abdomen and aids digestion.

TIPS Breathe normally and comfortably. Exaggerate the distending and contracting abdominal movements.

① Sit in half-lotus position. Place your fingers in a triangle around your lower abdomen. As you inhale, distend your abdomen as much as possible. As you exhale, contract your abdomen as much as you can. Perform 200 times.

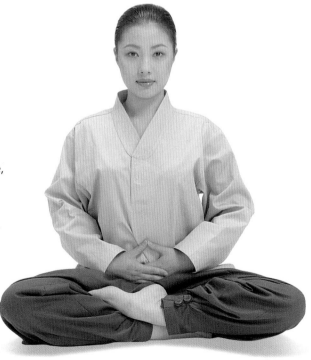

2. INTESTINE EXERCISES WITH RAISED HIPS

BENEFITS Stimulates the Stomach Meridian, helping to heal GI disorders and strengthen stomach muscles.

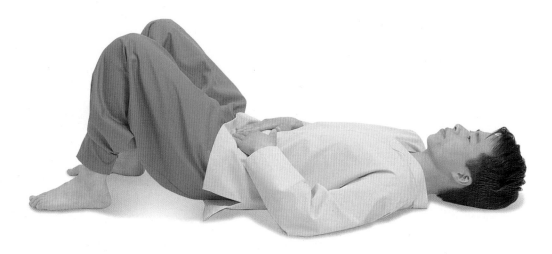

① Lie on your back and bend your knees with your feet flat on the floor, shoulder width apart. Form a triangle with your hands at the lower abdomen.

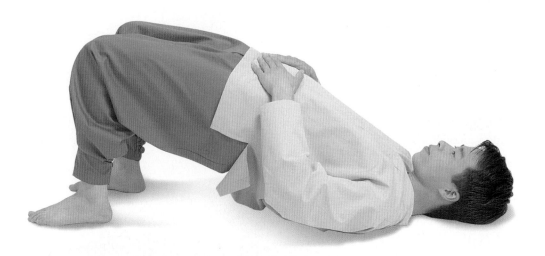

② Lift your hips off the floor, keeping your knees stable. Keeping your hips up, contract and distend the abdomen 200 times.

3. ARM MASSAGE

BENEFITS Maximizes Ki energy flow through the arms to strengthen heart, lungs, stomach, and intestines.

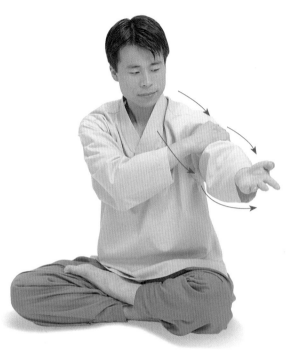

① Sit in a half-lotus position and extend your left arm in front of you with your thumb up. Massage from the shoulder to the elbow to the wrist. Proceed to the rest of the hand and massage under the pinky and up the bottom part of your arm toward your body, including your armpit. Then begin again at your shoulder. Perform in a continuous motion 36 times, alternating massaging the inner and outer parts of the arm.

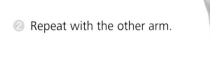

② Repeat with the other arm.

4. FOOT TO THIGH FORWARD BEND

BENEFITS Transports Ki energy accumulated in the lower abdomen to vital organs and the entire body. Helps to heal ulcers and to balance overproduction of acid secretions in the stomach. This exercise also alleviates sciatica, numbness in the hands and the feet, and shoulder pain and stimulates appetite.

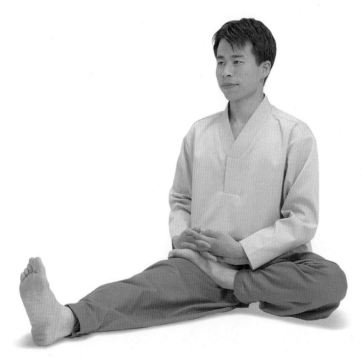

❶ Sit with your right leg extended in front of you, knee soft. Place your left foot comfortably on your right knee. Clasp your hands and place them on top of your left foot at the lower abdomen.

❷ Inhale. Bend from your hips while reaching your hands forward and clasping your fingers around your right foot.

❸ Continue to hold your breath for as long as you comfortably can. Exhale and return to the original posture.

❹ Repeat twice and then switch legs.

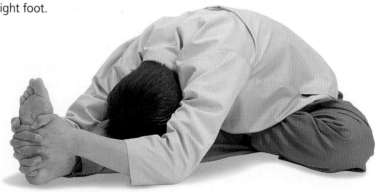

5. SEATED ANKLE ROTATION

BENEFITS Stimulates the Sp 2, Sp 3, and Sp 5 acupressure points in the foot. Strengthens a weak stomach and helps to alleviate discomfort from spasms in the stomach.

TIPS When performing this exercise, rotate only the ankle and the foot.

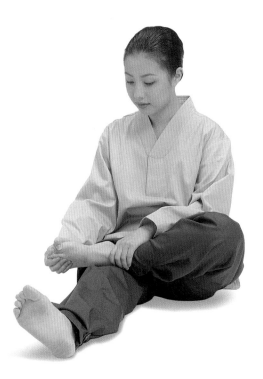

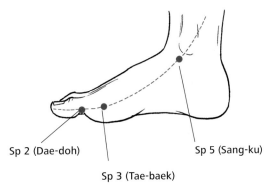

Sp 2 (Dae-doh)

Sp 5 (Sang-ku)

Sp 3 (Tae-baek)

❶ From a seated posture, extend your right leg with a soft knee and place your left foot on your right knee.

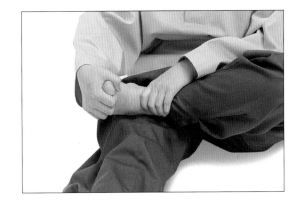

❷ Gently grasp your left ankle with your left hand. Grasp your toes with your right hand and push the toes backward to flex them. Alternate flexing and releasing them 4 times. Then, with your right hand still on your toes, proceed to rotate your ankle clockwise and counterclockwise in wide circles.

❸ Repeat with the other foot.

6. SITTING SPINAL TWIST

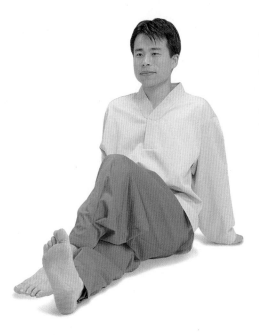

❶ Sit with your right leg extended, knee soft. Bend your left knee and cross the left foot over the right leg so it rests on the floor by your right knee.

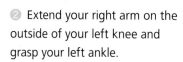

❷ Extend your right arm on the outside of your left knee and grasp your left ankle.

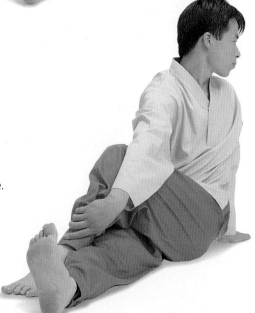

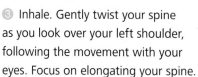

❸ Inhale. Gently twist your spine as you look over your left shoulder, following the movement with your eyes. Focus on elongating your spine.

❹ Exhale. Return to the original posture. Repeat twice to each side.

7. ROLLING BACK EXERCISE

BENEFITS Gently stimulates the spinal cord, strengthens the bone marrow and nervous system, and promotes optimal functioning of the vital organs.

TIPS Let your neck rhythmically follow the motion without pushing with your head. This is best performed on a lightly cushioned surface.

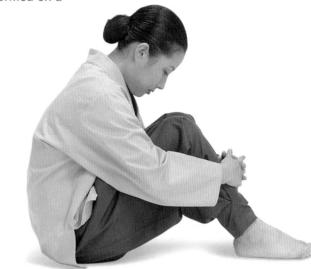

❶ Sit with your knees bent. Round your spine to form a *C* shape. Clasp your hands around your legs. Slightly lower your head. Relax your neck and your shoulders.

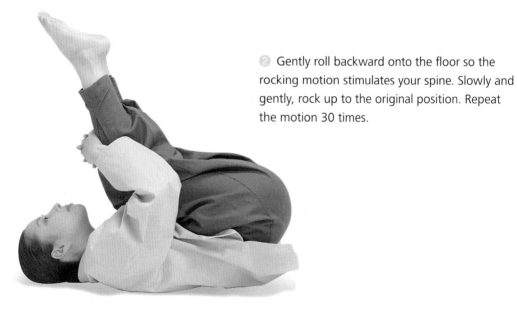

❷ Gently roll backward onto the floor so the rocking motion stimulates your spine. Slowly and gently, rock up to the original position. Repeat the motion 30 times.

8. LYING UPPER BODY TWIST

BENEFITS Stimulates 3 acupressure points: Lu 3, Ht 1, and PC 1, which in turn strengthens your heart and stomach.

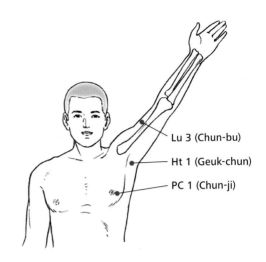

Lu 3 (Chun-bu)

Ht 1 (Geuk-chun)

PC 1 (Chun-ji)

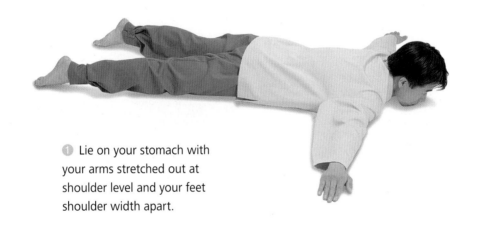

❶ Lie on your stomach with your arms stretched out at shoulder level and your feet shoulder width apart.

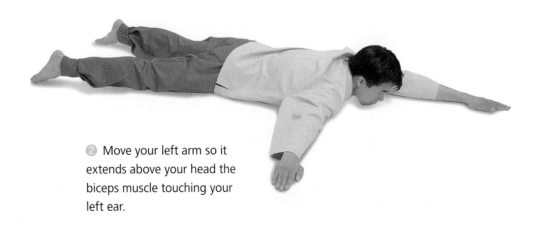

❷ Move your left arm so it extends above your head the biceps muscle touching your left ear.

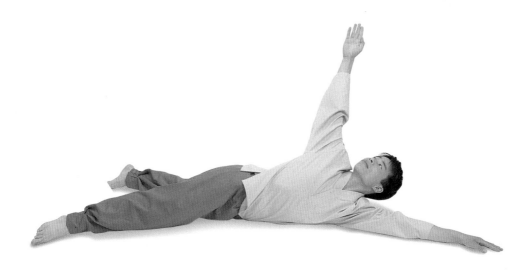

③ Inhale and lift your right arm toward the sky as you slowly turn and lift the right side of your upper body continue the motion of your right arm until the back of your hand touches the floor at shoulder level behind you. Keep your legs comfortably still and relax your neck and shoulders. Exhale and slowly return to the starting position.

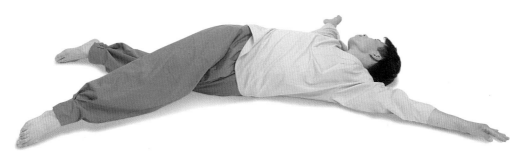

④ Repeat twice to the right and left sides.

9. POSTURE FOR STOMACH

BENEFITS Stimulates the Stomach Meridian, healing the stomach, gastrointestinal tract, and other related body parts.

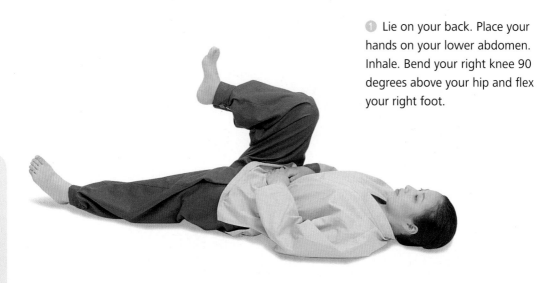

❶ Lie on your back. Place your hands on your lower abdomen. Inhale. Bend your right knee 90 degrees above your hip and flex your right foot.

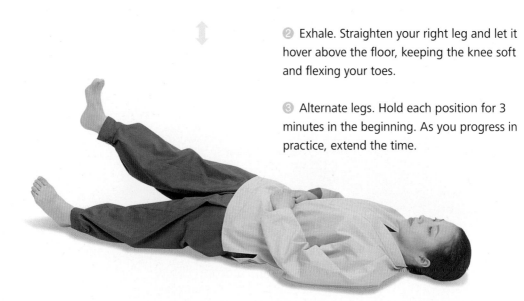

❷ Exhale. Straighten your right leg and let it hover above the floor, keeping the knee soft and flexing your toes.

❸ Alternate legs. Hold each position for 3 minutes in the beginning. As you progress in practice, extend the time.

10. PRESSING THE PALM

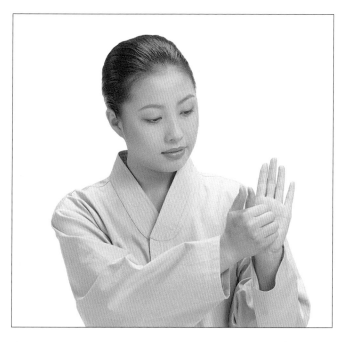

① Place 4 fingers of your left hand on the pad of your right hand. Curl the pad of your left hand around to the back of your right hand and squeeze. Continue to press for several seconds and release. Repeat several times for each hand.

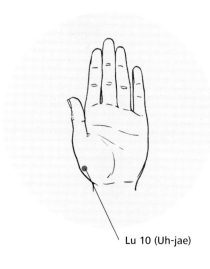

Lu 10 (Uh-jae)

② When you are very fatigued, your body becomes weak and your immune system can become compromised. The condition of the pad of the hand can reflect specific illnesses, such as pneumonia or bronchitis. The pad of the hand can feel hot to the touch. Examination of the pads can also reveal problems with other vital organs and symptoms affecting the gastrointestinal tract. Performing this exercise can assist in alleviating these symptoms.

LIVER DISORDERS

The liver is the largest organ in the body, and it filters and cleans the blood for your body to use. It is also a fat-burning organ. As toxicity builds up in the body, the liver must work harder, and its functioning is compromised. Predominant symptoms include tightness in the chest, digestive problems, headache, depression, dizziness, pain in the joints, sleeping disorders, dry skin, eczema, pallid and tired-looking skin, edema, redness in the palms of the hands and tips of the fingers, nausea, fatigue, abdominal pain in the upper right quadrant, and difficulty in anger and irritability management. This can create a vicious cycle that blocks heat energy in the liver, resulting in further damage to the liver and an increase in symptoms.

The exercises recommended in this section stimulate the Liver Meridian, which warms the body, oxygenates the blood, and circulates Ki energy to vital organs. The resultant increase in perspiration releases toxins, and abdominal breathing synchronizes the abdomen with the diaphragm, which in turn stimulates the liver function.

BACK BEND CHEST OPENING (P. 49)

BENEFITS Stimulates the thyroid, kidney, liver, and pancreas.

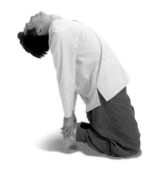

LIFTING LEGS OVER HEAD (P. 62)

BENEFITS Stimulates autonomic nervous system and vital organs, such as the heart, liver, and spleen.

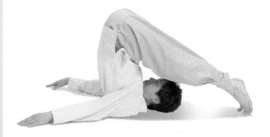

PELVIC REALIGNMENT (P. 100)

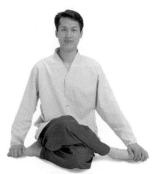

1. EXPANDING CHEST WITH ARM RAISING

TIPS Stand with your legs straight and knees soft.

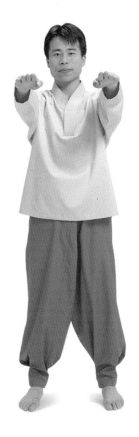

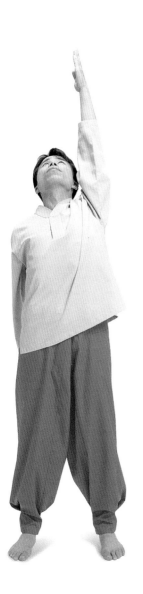

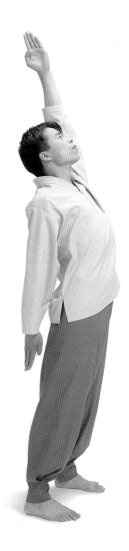

① Extend arms in front of you so they are parallel to the floor with your palms down. Relax your neck and shoulders.

② Inhale. Raise your left arm up slowly with your palm facing inside. Follow the movement of this hand with your eyes. Simultaneously reach down and behind you with your right arm, fingers extended and palm turned inside. Focus on expanding your chest.

③ Exhale. Return to STEP 1.

④ Alternate arms. Repeat 3 times.

2. STRUTTING BIRD BALANCE

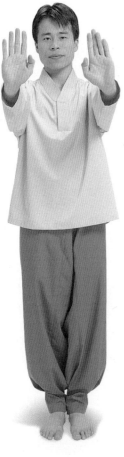

LIVER DISORDERS

① Stand with your feet together. Extend your arms at shoulder level in front of you, wrists flexed.

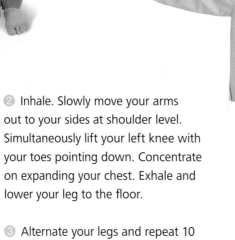

② Inhale. Slowly move your arms out to your sides at shoulder level. Simultaneously lift your left knee with your toes pointing down. Concentrate on expanding your chest. Exhale and lower your leg to the floor.

③ Alternate your legs and repeat 10 times. Perform this exercise very slowly.

3. SIDE BEND WITH FLEXED WRISTS

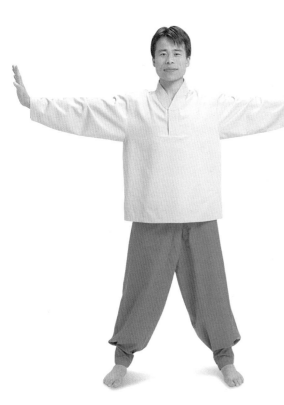

① Stand with your legs shoulder width apart. Extend your arms out to the sides at shoulder level with flexed wrists.

② Inhale. Raise your right hand up over your head, following the movement with your eyes. Wrap your left hand around to the right side and bend to the left with your right palm facing the sky. Exhale and return to the beginning posture.

③ Switch hands. Inhale and bend to the other side. Repeat 10 times.

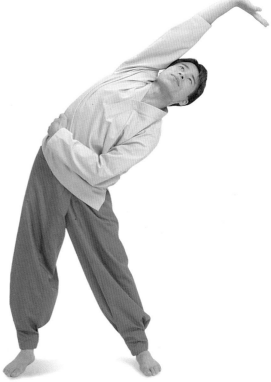

4. UPPER BODY TWIST

BENEFITS Releases stagnant energy from the shoulders, chest, and arms. Strengthens the lungs and liver.

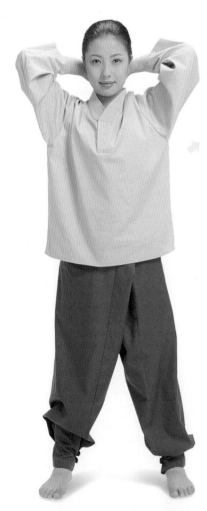

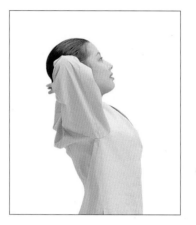

❷ Hold your breath while lifting and supporting your neck, and tilt your head back to look at the sky. Focus upon your ribs and spine. Exhale and return to STEP 1.

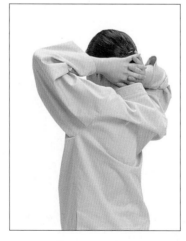

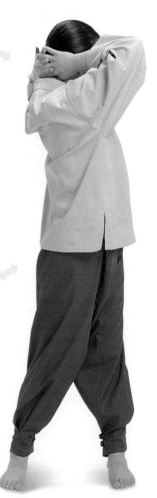

❶ Stand with your feet shoulder width apart. Inhale and interlace your fingers behind your neck. Use both hands to press the back of the neck, lifting and supporting it.

❸ Turn to the left and right very slowly 10 times.

5. CLAMSHELL SIT-UP

BENEFIT Enhances liver function in a short period of time.

TIPS Keep your legs and toes straight but with soft knees.

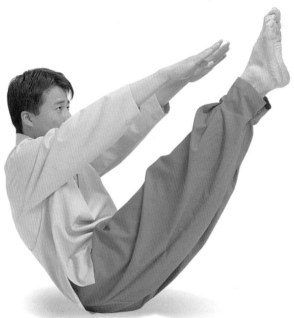

❶ Lie on your back with your feet together and arms at your sides. Simultaneously raise your upper body and legs so only your hips stay on the floor. Aim your fingers to touch your toes. If touching your toes is difficult for you in the beginning, you can alternately touch your ankles.

LIVER DISORDERS

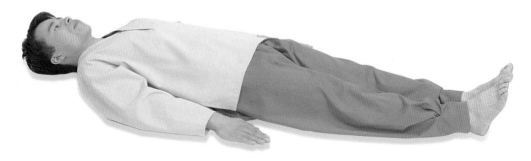

❷ Return to starting position and relax for 10 seconds. Repeat 5 times.

6. TWISTING KNEE TOUCH

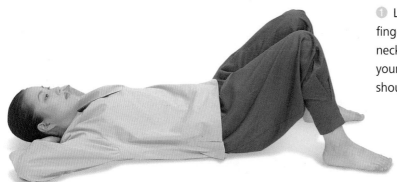

① Lie on your back with your fingers interlaced behind your neck. Bend your knees so your feet are flat on the floor, shoulder width apart.

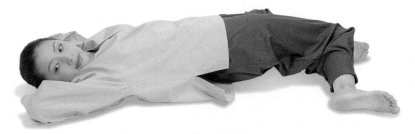

② Inhale. While keeping your shoulders still, turn your head to the right side and simultaneously move both knees to the left to touch the floor.

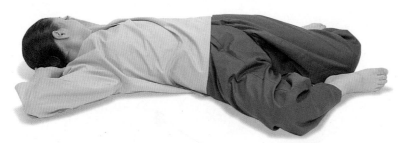

③ Exhale. Return to STEP 1. Now turn your head to the left side while simultaneously moving both knees to the right side and touching the floor. Repeat 3 times, alternating to the left and right sides.

7. SEATED SIDE BEND

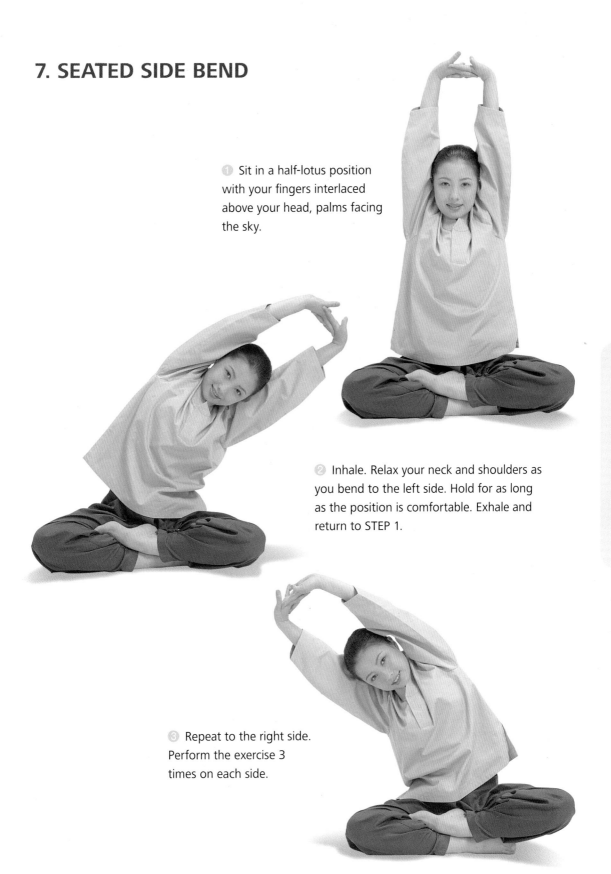

① Sit in a half-lotus position with your fingers interlaced above your head, palms facing the sky.

② Inhale. Relax your neck and shoulders as you bend to the left side. Hold for as long as the position is comfortable. Exhale and return to STEP 1.

③ Repeat to the right side. Perform the exercise 3 times on each side.

8. BRIDGE POSTURE

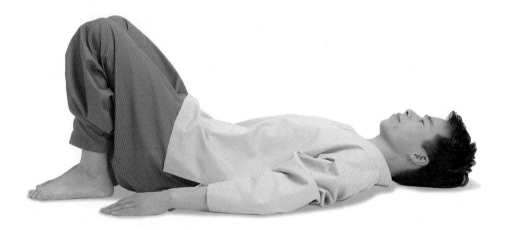

① Lie on your back and bend your knees
so your heels rest on the floor close to
your hips.

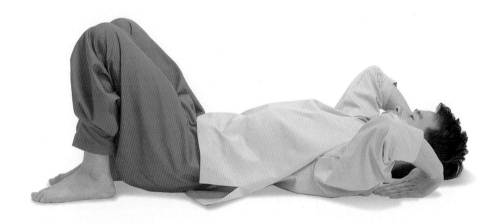

② Place your hands palm down on
either side of your head with your fingers
pointing toward your feet.

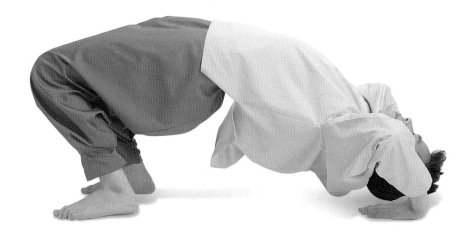

③ Inhale. Press your hands and feet into the floor while simultaneously raising your shoulders and hips and then your head so your body forms an arch. Do not strain to reach this position.

④ Hold this posture for as long as you comfortably can.

⑤ Relax, exhale, and return to STEP 2. Repeat 3 times.

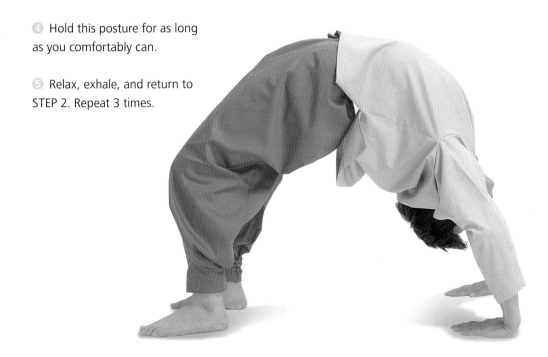

9. CROSSING LEG TO TOUCH FINGERS

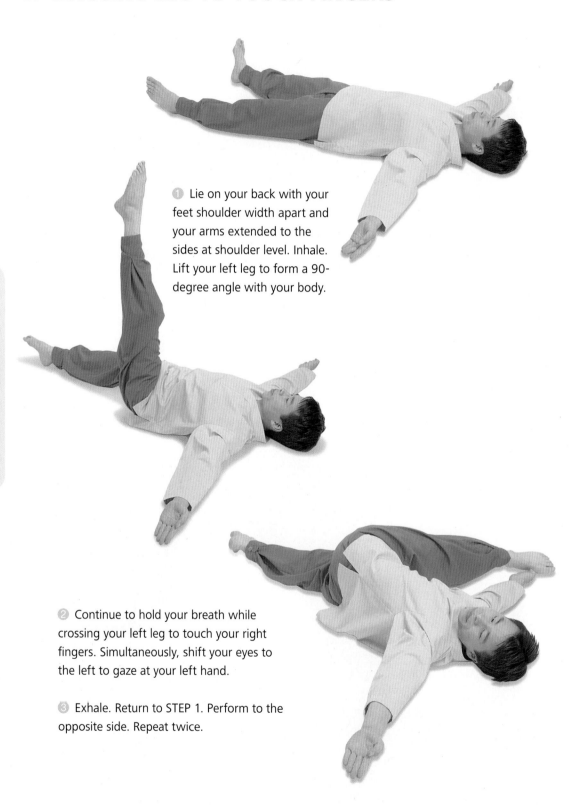

❶ Lie on your back with your feet shoulder width apart and your arms extended to the sides at shoulder level. Inhale. Lift your left leg to form a 90-degree angle with your body.

❷ Continue to hold your breath while crossing your left leg to touch your right fingers. Simultaneously, shift your eyes to the left to gaze at your left hand.

❸ Exhale. Return to STEP 1. Perform to the opposite side. Repeat twice.

10. SENDING KI ENERGY TO EYES

BENEFITS Improves liver conditions by exercising the eyes, as the condition of the eyes is related to the functioning of the liver.

TIP Keep your eyes open during this exercise.

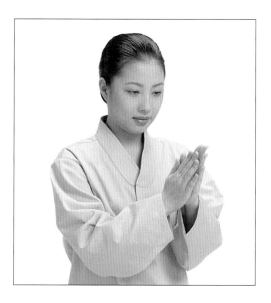

❶ Place your palms together. Inhale deeply through the abdomen. Rub your palms together 50 times.

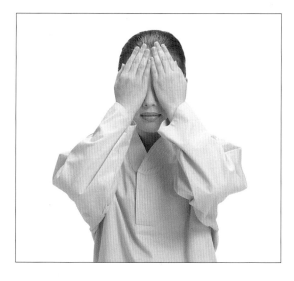

❷ Place both of your hands over your eyes with the center of the palms closest to your eyes.

❸ Exhale. Rotate your eyeballs, looking up and down, clockwise and counterclockwise , and to either side 10 times each.

11. SIDE TO SIDE LEG LIFTS

TIPS If you have back problems, perform this exercise with caution. If you experience any pressure in your head while your legs are raised to a 90-degree angle, you may want to elevate your head very slightly while performing this exercise.

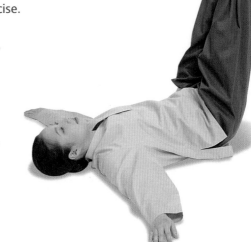

① Lie on your back with your arms extended to your sides at shoulder level. Keeping your legs together with soft knees, raise them to a 90-degree angle above your hips.

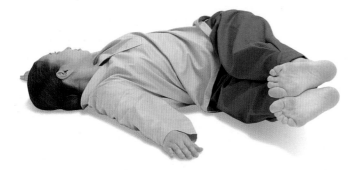

② Inhale. Bring both of your legs to the right and gently touch the floor. Gaze in the direction of your left hand. Hold for 2-3 seconds. As you progress in this exercise, you will be able to touch your right hand with your feet.

③ Exhale and slowly brings your legs back to a 90-degree angle, as in STEP 1.

④ Lower your feet slowly to the left side while gazing to the right. Repeat 5 times.

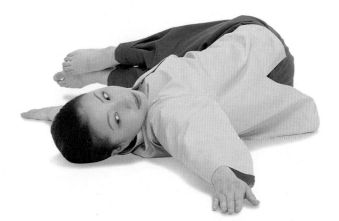

12. LIVER ENERGIZER

BENEFITS Stimulates and strengthens the liver while relieving fatigue. Also strengthens the knee joints to prevent arthritis and strengthens the lower extremities and the lower abdomen.

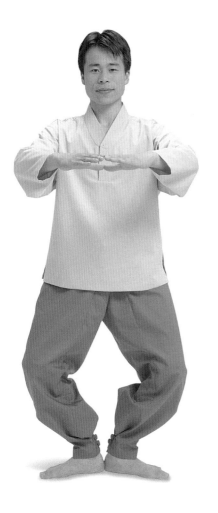

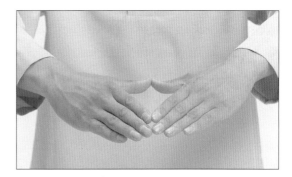

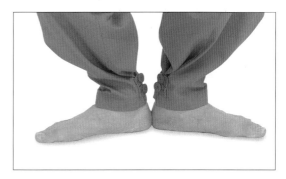

① Stand with your heels together and your toes pointing out at a 180-degree angle and your knees bent. Keep your spine straight with your neck and shoulders relaxed. Place your arms in front of your chest with your palms down, thumbs and index fingers touching to form a triangle.

② Hold this posture for as long as you are comfortable. Accompany this exercise with abdominal breathing as you progress in your practice.

DIARRHEA

When the large intestine, or colon, functions properly, it absorbs liquid from the small intestine's waste, providing the body with nutrients before the waste passes from the body. Diarrhea impairs the large intestine's ability to absorb liquid due to either a secretion from the bowel that blocks absorption or the swift passage of waste through the bowel, which leaves no time for proper absorption of nutrients.

Under normal circumstances, diarrhea subsides in two to three days. However, if symptoms persist, particularly if they are accompanied by a high fever and severe pain in the abdomen, then a more serious condition could be present, warranting medical attention. Diarrhea can be generated and exacerbated by the presence of stress as well as by erratic eating habits. It is helpful to stimulate the feet, palms, and lower abdomen with massage to improve the digestive and absorption processes.

SITTING FORWARD BEND (P. 50)

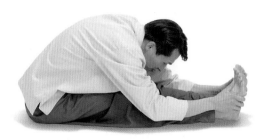

LIFTING LEGS OVER HEAD (P. 62)

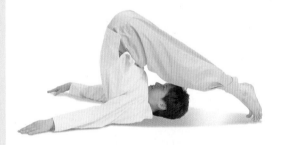

1. LOWER BACK ACUPRESSURE

TIP It is important to focus on expanding your chest to relax your body while performing this exercise.

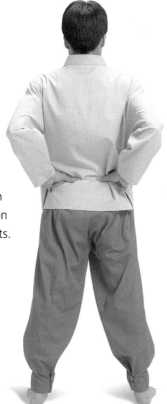

Bl 25
(Dae-jang-yu)

Bl 27
(So-jang-yu)

Bl 25 acupressure points are located about two inches to either side of the fourth and fifth lumbar vertebrae. The Bl 27 acupressure points are about one inch below the Bl 25 points.

❶ Stand with your feet parallel and shoulder width apart. Place your thumbs on the Bl 25 acupressure points.

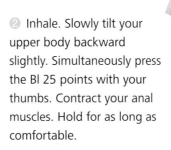

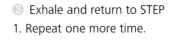

❷ Inhale. Slowly tilt your upper body backward slightly. Simultaneously press the Bl 25 points with your thumbs. Contract your anal muscles. Hold for as long as comfortable.

❸ Exhale and return to STEP 1. Repeat one more time.

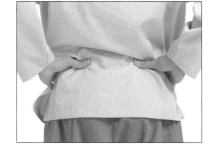

2. LOWER BACK PATTING

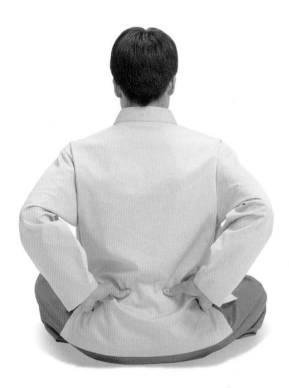

① Sit in a half-lotus position. Place your thumbs on the Bl 27 (So-jang-yu) acupressure points, and then press and massage them until you generate heat energy in the area. Follow with rubbing with a quick motion in the vicinity of these acupressure points.

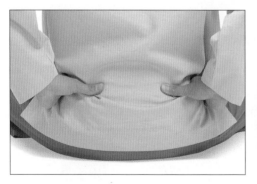

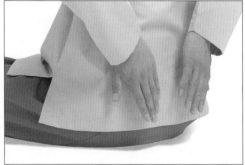

② Repeat STEPs 1 and 2 with the Bl 25 (Dae-jang-yu) points.

3. HIP LIFTS

BENEFIT Stops mild diarrhea.

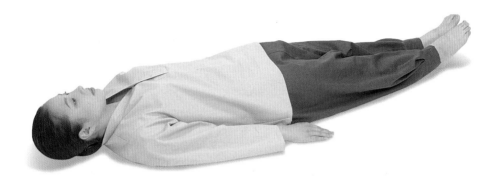

❶ Lie on your back with your feet together and your hands by your side.

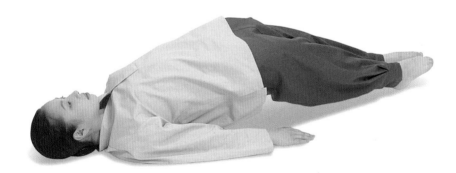

❷ Inhale. Gently raise your waist, hips, and back to support your body while your hands, arms, and heels are still on the floor.

❸ Hold this posture for 10 seconds. Exhale and gently lower your body to the floor. Repeat 5 times.

CONSTIPATION

Constipation occurs when bowel movements become difficult or infrequent. It is usually caused by inadequate water intake, insufficient fiber in the diet, a disruption of regular diet or routine, immobility, or prolonged stress.

Seniors are particularly vulnerable to constipation. As we age, peristaltic movements are not as efficient and waste accumulates in the intestine for a prolonged period of time. All water and moisture are absorbed, adversely affecting the intestine's ability to pass the waste from the body. Due to hormonal changes in the menstrual cycle, which impact the secretion of the hormones relating to the peristaltic motions of the large intestine, women experience constipation more often than men. To prevent constipation, it is imperative to exercise regularly; it is particularly important to maintain strong abdominal muscles.

When you perform the meridian exercises in this section, coordinate them with abdominal breathing and synchronous movements of expanding and contracting the abdomen. Intestine exercise is the most powerful and efficient way to prevent and relieve constipation.

INTESTINE EXERCISE (P. 26)

TIPS Concentrate on expansion and contraction of the lower abdomen.

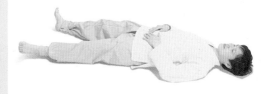

SIT-UP (P. 106)

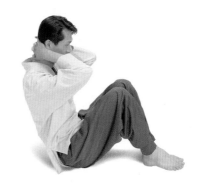

TAILBONE TAPPING (P. 265)

BENEFITS Enhances the autonomic nervous system and efficient peristaltic movements.

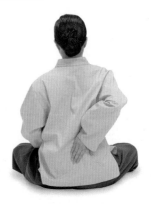

1. FISH EXERCISE

BENEFITS Strengthens spinal nerves and enriches blood circulation, keeps the intestines in their proper placement and shape, and relieves constipation.

TIPS Synchronize your movements so that your upper and lower body move in the same direction. Keep your feet together as you perform these movements.

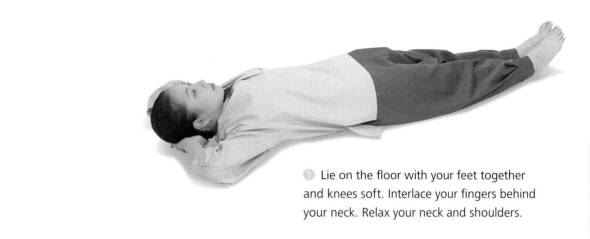

① Lie on the floor with your feet together and knees soft. Interlace your fingers behind your neck. Relax your neck and shoulders.

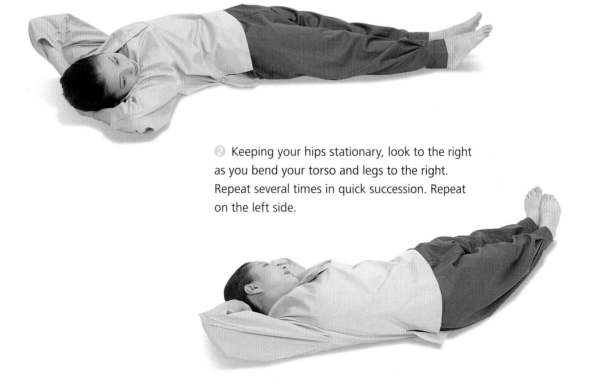

② Keeping your hips stationary, look to the right as you bend your torso and legs to the right. Repeat several times in quick succession. Repeat on the left side.

2. LEG LIFT VARIATION

① Lie in a semireclining posture with your elbows on the floor and your hands supporting your waist.

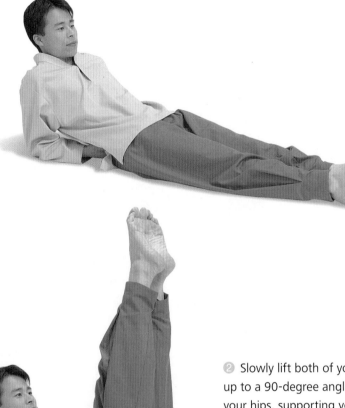

② Slowly lift both of your legs up to a 90-degree angle above your hips, supporting your body with your elbows. Relax your neck and your shoulders.

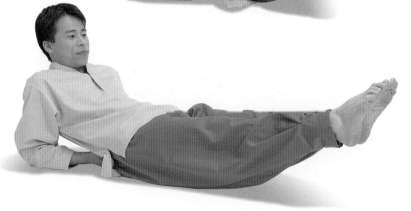

③ Slowly lower your legs without touching the floor. Repeat 10 times.

3. LYING KNEE PULL

BENEFITS Relieves constipation. Strengthens women's reproductive system.

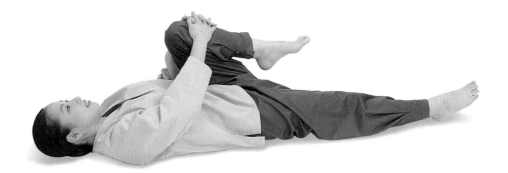

1 Lie on your back and bend your left knee toward your chest. Interlace your fingers around the shin of your left leg. Extend your right leg straight out in front, maintaining a soft knee.

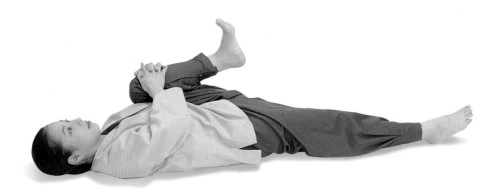

2 Inhale. Flex your left foot. Pull your left knee as close to your chest as you can.

3 Exhale. Return to STEP 1. Change legs and proceed. Repeat 3 times with each leg.

4. ABDOMINAL SQUEEZE

① Lie on your back with your knees pulled toward your chest. Interlace your fingers around the shins of your legs.

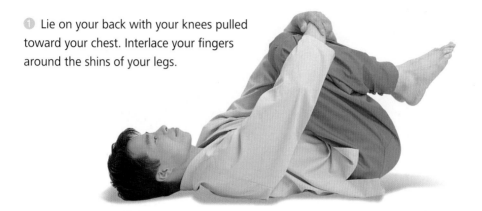

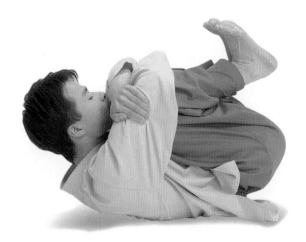

② Inhale. Gently pull your knees to your chest, while simultaneously lifting your head to touch your knees. Focus on your lower abdomen.

③ Exhale. Slowly lower your legs, knees bent, and place your feet on the floor. Rest your arms by your side with your palms facing the floor. Relax your body.

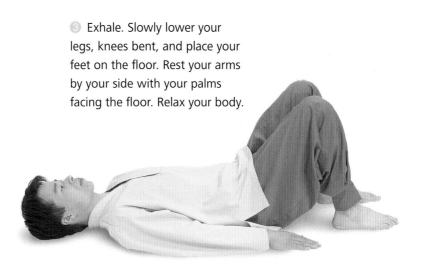

④ Inhale. Gently lift your lower abdomen to the sky as far as you comfortably can. Exhale and relax. Repeat 3 times.

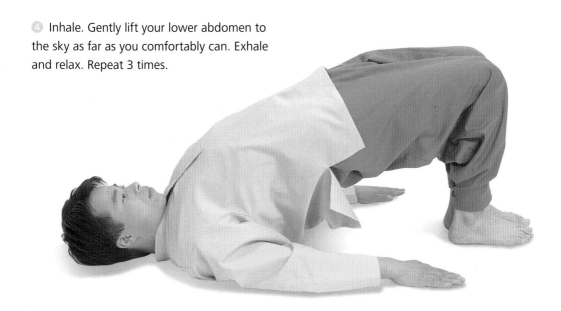

5. ROLLING BOW POSTURE

BENEFITS Realigns the spine and strengthens peristaltic movement of the intestines, thereby healing problems with constipation. Releases toxins as it aids the elimination process.

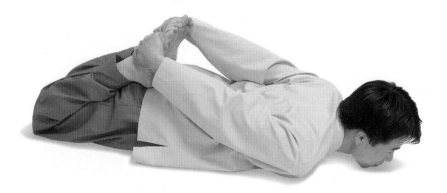

❶ Lie on your stomach with your chin touching the floor. Bend your knees and lift your feet toward your head.

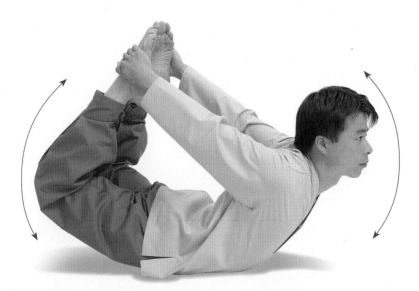

❷ Grasp your feet with your hands. Gently lift your head, upper body, and knees while holding your feet, forming a bow posture. Only your lower abdomen will be in contact with the floor. Begin a rocking motion backward and forward.

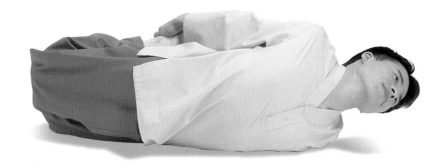

❸ Slowly turn onto your side and rock to the right and left.

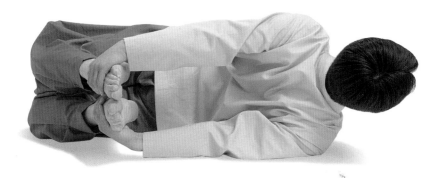

❹ Repeat the above steps, but this time, perform your motions very slowly and comfortably to thoroughly stimulate your internal organs.

6. TWISTING SOLE SLAP

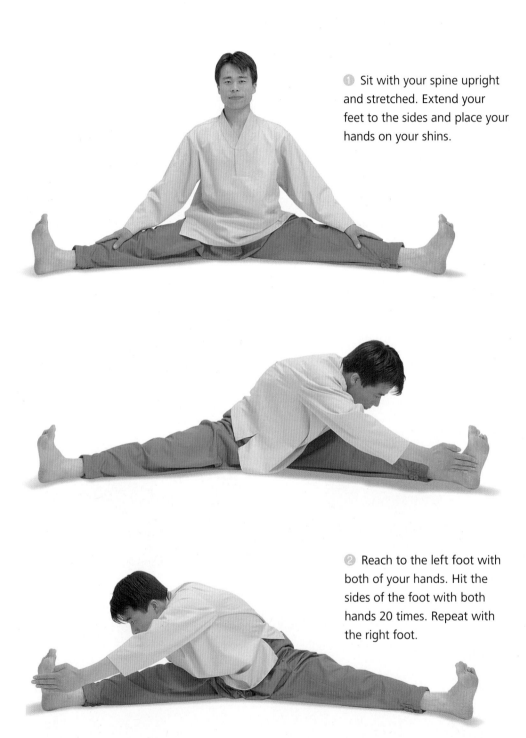

❶ Sit with your spine upright and stretched. Extend your feet to the sides and place your hands on your shins.

❷ Reach to the left foot with both of your hands. Hit the sides of the foot with both hands 20 times. Repeat with the right foot.

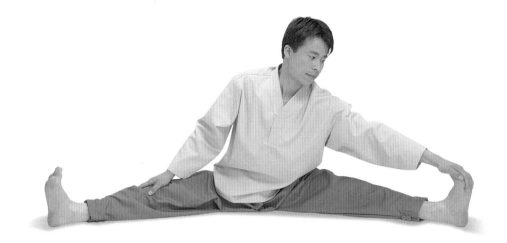

③ Place your left hand on your left toes and your right hand on your right thigh. Bend from the waist while bringing your right hand over your head to the left foot. Glide your left hand to the heel while placing your right hand around the toes. Hold for as long as comfortable while focusing on the bending of your waist. Then return to the starting position.

④ Repeat twice on each side.

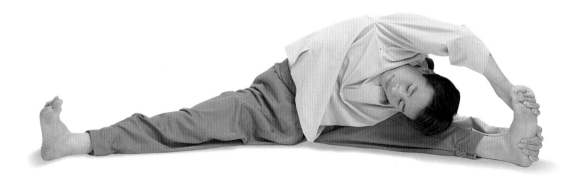

HEMORRHOIDS

Hemorrhoids occur when the blood vessels around the circumference of the anus become swollen due to stagnant blood in the area. When you sit or stand in the same posture for extended periods of time, pressure around the anus is increased, impeding circulation. If you also suffer from constipation, the problem may be exacerbated by the extreme pressure.

It is important to maintain warmth in the lower abdomen, take measures to ensure healthy elimination patterns, and avoid sitting on a cold surface. Hemorrhoids are often caused by faulty intestinal functioning. Even if one undergoes a hemorrhoidectomy, one can still suffer from a re-occurrence of hemorrhoids if the problem of the intestines is not resolved.

The exercises recommended here encourage healthy shunting of blood flow to the anal area, thereby mitigating the swelling that causes hemorrhoids. Practicing these meridian exercises will strengthen the intestines as well as alleviate constipation.

ANAL CONTRACTING EXERCISE (P. 27)

BENEFITS Prevents hemorrhoid formation and treats hemorrhoids when they occur. Eliminates anal swelling by enhancing Ki and blood circulation around the anus. You can practice this exercise anytime and anyplace.

BICYCLE EXERCISE (P. 140)

BENEFITS Strengthens lower extremities, muscles and nerves around the perineum, and reproductive glands. Strengthens Ki and blood circulation. Prevents and treats hemorrhoids. Releases fatigue from the head and the lower extremities as it enhances stamina.

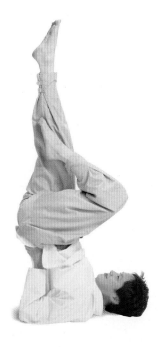

1. CROWN TAPPING

BENEFITS Alleviates pain associated with hemorrhoids by stimulating the acupressure point on the top of the head.

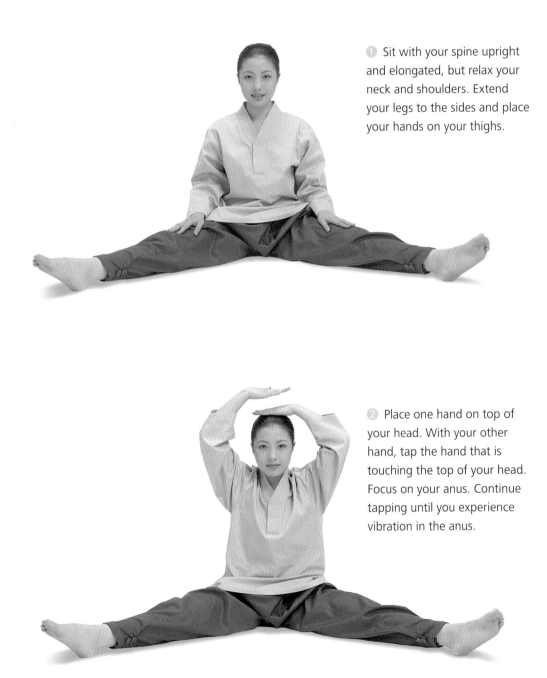

❶ Sit with your spine upright and elongated, but relax your neck and shoulders. Extend your legs to the sides and place your hands on your thighs.

❷ Place one hand on top of your head. With your other hand, tap the hand that is touching the top of your head. Focus on your anus. Continue tapping until you experience vibration in the anus.

2. HIP LIFT WITH ANKLE HOLD

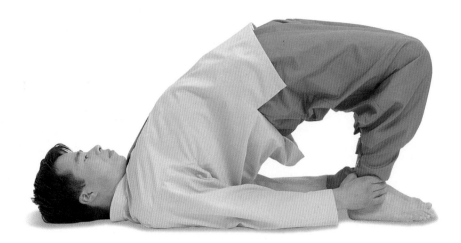

❶ Lie on your back with your heels placed close to your buttocks. Grasp your ankles. Inhale and gently lift your hips up so your weight is on your shoulders and heels. Contract your anus and hold this posture. Focus on your lower abdomen.

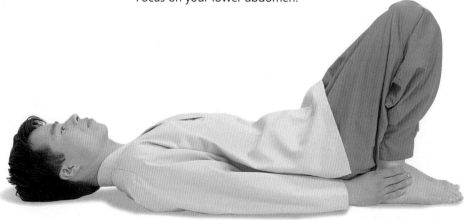

❷ Exhale. Slowly lower your hips. Repeat 5 times.

3. STANDING KNEE PULL

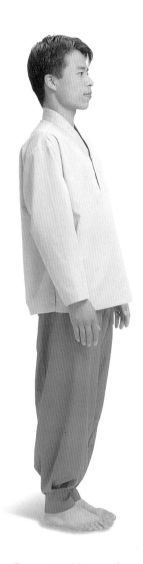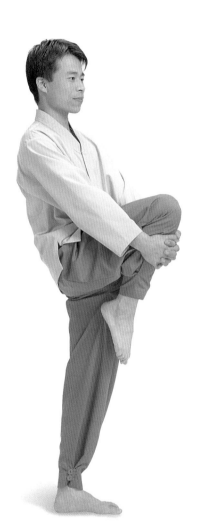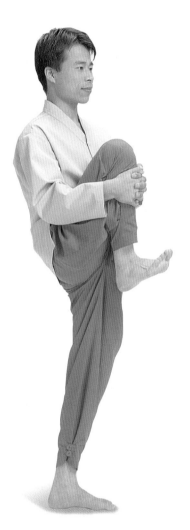

① Stand with your feet together and your spine straight. Inhale. Interlace your fingers around the shin of one leg and pull your knee toward your chest.

② Flex your foot so your toes point toward the sky. Align your neck and back.

③ Exhale. Release your fingers and return to the standing position with both of your feet on the floor. Repeat with your other leg. Perform 3 times with each leg.

KIDNEY DISORDERS

A kidney malfunction can cause bloating in the abdomen and legs, a feeling of heaviness in the body, and cold sweats during sleep. You may feel a preference to sleep on your stomach. Upon awakening, you might experience swelling and discomfort around the circumference of your waist.

Abdominal breathing treats kidney disorders by stimulating the kidneys as they move up and down, facilitating Ki energy and blood circulation to this organ.

The kidneys control the vital energy in the lower abdomen. As you focus your attention on your Myung-moon acupressure point and breathe through this point as part of abdominal breathing, it will amplify the energy in the lower abdomen. As you continue to practice this breathing, the kidney is less burdened by filtering the blood and excreting toxins from the body. The recommended meridian exercises in this chapter will stimulate the Urinary Bladder Meridian and enhance kidney functioning.

CIRCULATION EXERCISE (P. 24)

TIPS Extend knees, arms, and elbows. If your neck is uncomfortable, you may place a wooden pillow under it for support.

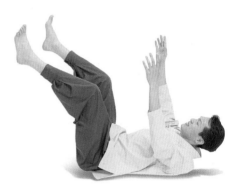

UPPER BODY LIFT (P. 48)

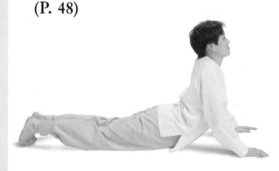

SITTING FORWARD BEND (P. 50)

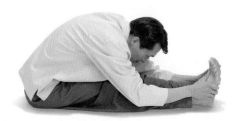

LIFTING LEGS OVER HEAD (P. 62)

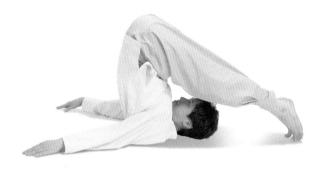

RAISING HANDS (P. 69)

TIPS As you tilt backward, follow the movement with the gaze of your eyes. If you experience dizziness, your body condition is weak, or you are an elder, minimize your tilting. Gaze with your eyes toward the horizon, rather than toward your fingertips. Place your weight on the back of the right foot, toes, lower abdomen, and waist.

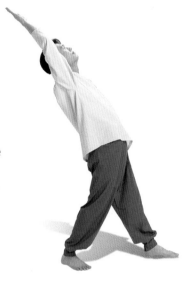

SOLE PATTING
(P. 39)

FACE-DOWN TOE
TOUCH (P. 102)

TIPS The Ki 1 (Yong-chun) acupressure points on the soles of the feet are connected to the kidney. It is helpful to practice applying pressure with a wooden stick or your fingers to stimulate the Yong-chun point in the morning for about 5 minutes.

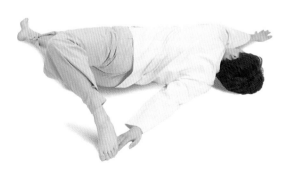

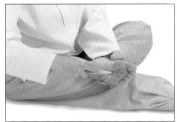

1. KIDNEY ACUPRESSURE

Bl 52 (Ji-shil)

Bl 23 (Shin-yu)

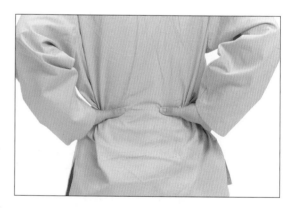

• Bl 23 acupressure points are located on either side of the second lumbar vertebrae.

• Bl 52 acupressure points are located on either side of the second lumbar vertebrae and about one and one half inches to the outside of the Bl 23 points.

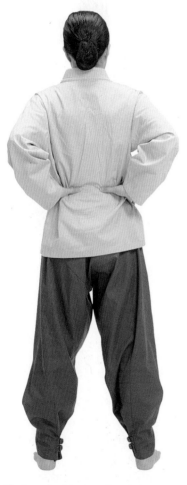

① Stand with your feet shoulder width apart. Place your thumbs on the Bl 23 (Shin-yu) points.

② Inhale while you press the Bl 23 points with your thumbs. Gently tilt your upper body backward.

③ Hold your breath as you press with your thumbs and focus on your waist.

④ Release your thumbs. Exhale. Repeat twice. Then perform the same exercise with the Bl 52 (Ji-shil) points.

2. KIDNEY STIMULATION

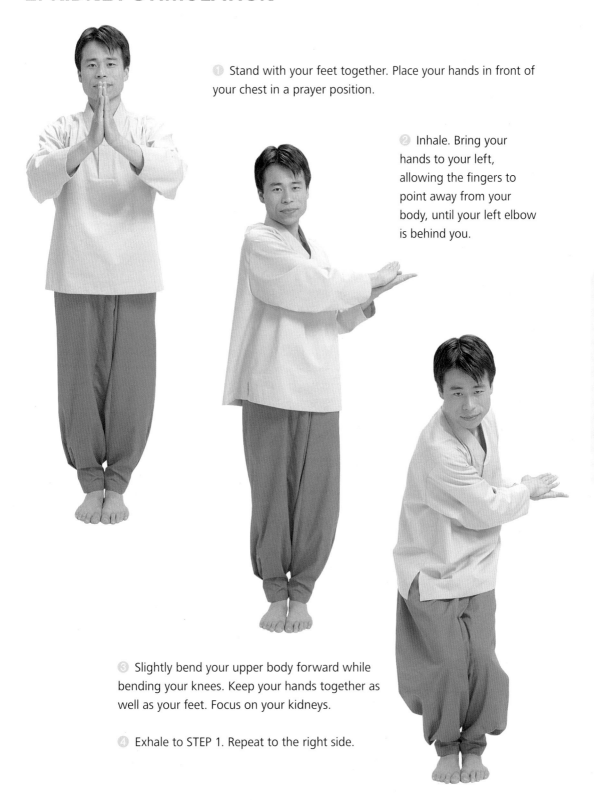

① Stand with your feet together. Place your hands in front of your chest in a prayer position.

② Inhale. Bring your hands to your left, allowing the fingers to point away from your body, until your left elbow is behind you.

③ Slightly bend your upper body forward while bending your knees. Keep your hands together as well as your feet. Focus on your kidneys.

④ Exhale to STEP 1. Repeat to the right side.

3. LEG LIFT

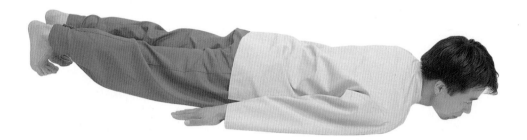

① Lie on your stomach. Place your hands at your sides with palms facing down and toes flexed.

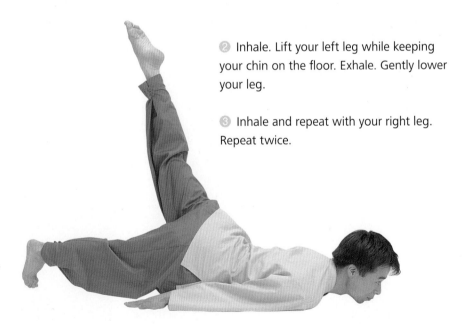

② Inhale. Lift your left leg while keeping your chin on the floor. Exhale. Gently lower your leg.

③ Inhale and repeat with your right leg. Repeat twice.

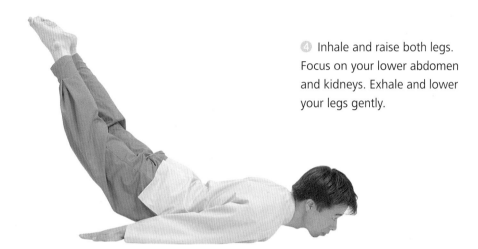

④ Inhale and raise both legs. Focus on your lower abdomen and kidneys. Exhale and lower your legs gently.

4. KIDNEY MASSAGE

BENEFITS Releases stagnant energy from the kidneys, enhancing their function. Also cools the lower extremities. Kidney massage performed directly on the skin without clothes is ideal.

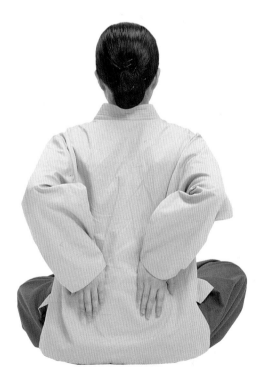

Inhale. Rub your hands together until they are hot. Press your hands on your kidneys, fingers pointing down, and massage in an up-and-down motion.

5. ANKLE ACUPRESSURE

BENEFITS Stimulates acupressure points to enhance stamina and infuse energy in the Dahn-jon, which can reverse roughness in the heel pads and regenerate elasticity in the area.

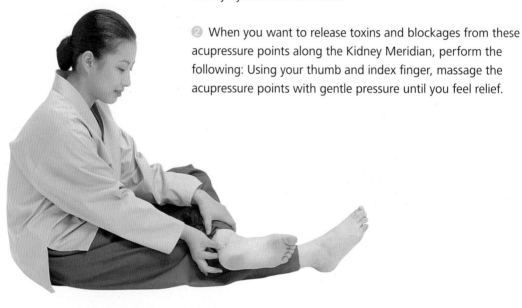

① Five acupressure points—Ki 3, Ki 4, Ki 5, Ki 6, and Ki 12 —are located in the inner ankle area and compose the Kidney Meridian. When there are blockages along this meridian, kidney dysfunction can occur.

② When you want to release toxins and blockages from these acupressure points along the Kidney Meridian, perform the following: Using your thumb and index finger, massage the acupressure points with gentle pressure until you feel relief.

KIDNEY DISORDERS

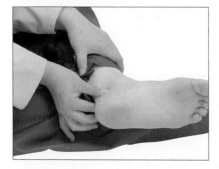

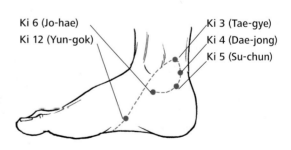

Ki 6 (Jo-hae)
Ki 12 (Yun-gok)
Ki 3 (Tae-gye)
Ki 4 (Dae-jong)
Ki 5 (Su-chun)

6. ABDOMINAL BREATHING

BENEFITS Accumulates heat energy in the Dahn-jon and kidneys to enhance kidney function.

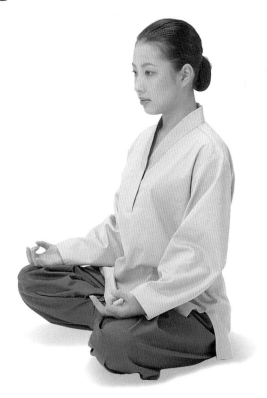

❶ Sit in a half-lotus position with your hands resting comfortably on the tops of your legs, palms up. When you inhale, focus on the GV 4 (Myung-moon) point becoming warmer. The GV 4 point is located directly behind the navel in front of the spine, near the kidneys.

❷ Notice the gentle expansion of the abdomen. When you exhale, slowly pull the abdomen inward. Again, inhale and push the abdomen gently out and down at a 45-degree angle.

❸ As you inhale, focus on the flow of Ki energy through the GV 4 point and downward toward the Dahn-jon. Visualize the GV 4 point as the opening in the body and the abdomen as a balloon collecting the Ki energy. This will foster accumulation of Ki energy in the Dahn-jon. As the kidneys and the Dahn-jon become warmer, water energy is activated to enhance kidney function.

GV 4 (Myung-moon)

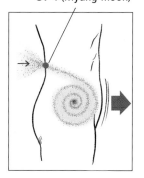

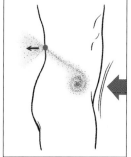

When you inhale, the abdomen expands.

When you exhale, the abdomen contracts.

LEG SWEEP (P. 97)

BENEFITS Helps chronic lumbago, waist, and lower extremities; promotes a feeling of vitality.

BLADDER INFECTION

Bladder infections occur when a virus or bacterium penetrates the bladder membranes and moves through the urethra to the urinary tract. The infection can recur and become chronic. People who sit for long periods of time are more susceptible to infection because of compression of the bladder. Women are more prone to contracting urinary tract infections (UTIs) due to short urinary tracts.

Urinating regularly is the most important method to fight and prevent UTIs. Hydrating well can help to flush troublesome organisms from the body, and urination reduces the possibility of viruses and bacteria infecting the urinary tract.

The exercises in this section, as well as abdominal breathing, assist in the accumulation of Ki energy in the lower abdomen, thereby boosting the immune system and expediting recovery from infection of the bladder. Urinate just before and rigth after these exercises.

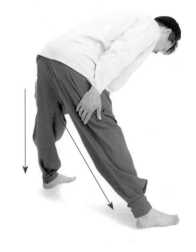

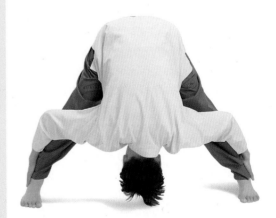

1. LEG SWINGS

BENEFITS Helps chronic lumbago, waist, and lower extremities; promotes a feeling of vitality.

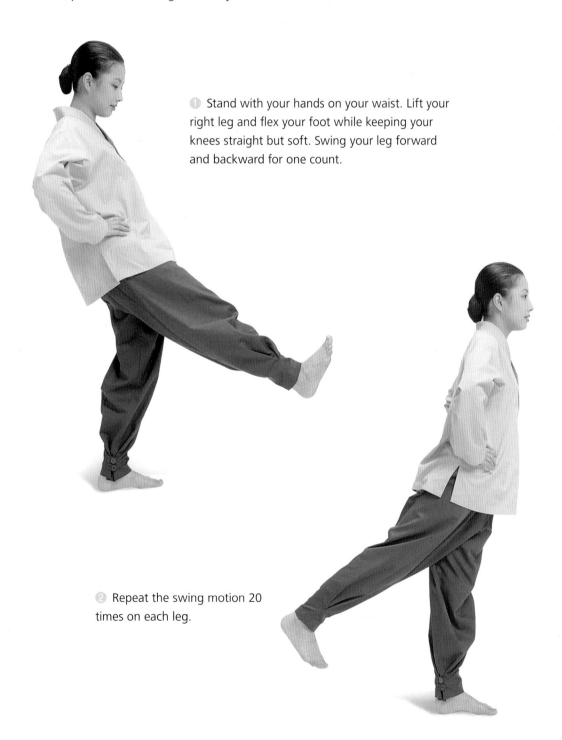

❶ Stand with your hands on your waist. Lift your right leg and flex your foot while keeping your knees straight but soft. Swing your leg forward and backward for one count.

❷ Repeat the swing motion 20 times on each leg.

2. HEEL DROP EXERCISE

TIP Focus on landing on your heels with the weight of your whole body.

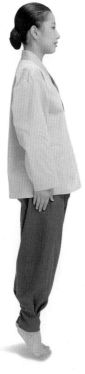

① Stand with your feet together and your arms at your sides. Inhale. Raise yourself on your toes.

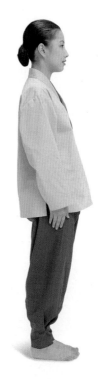

② Exhale and drop your weight back on your heels, exaggerating the drop using the weight of your whole body.

3. RAISED LEG FOOT TAPPING

① Lie on your back with your arms extended to the sides. Lift your legs above your hips 90 degrees and flex your feet, but keep your knees soft.

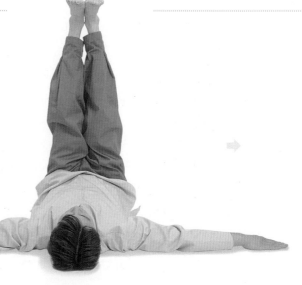

4. FOOT TO FACE LEG STRETCH

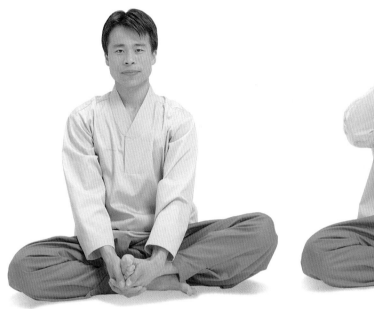
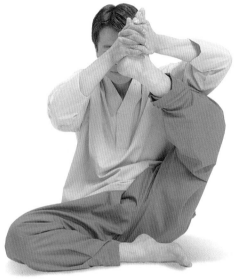

1. While sitting with your legs crossed, interlace your fingers around your left foot.

2. Inhale and gently bring the sole of your foot toward your face. Hold for as long as is comfortable. Exhale and lower your foot. Perform the same motions with your right foot. Repeat 3 times.

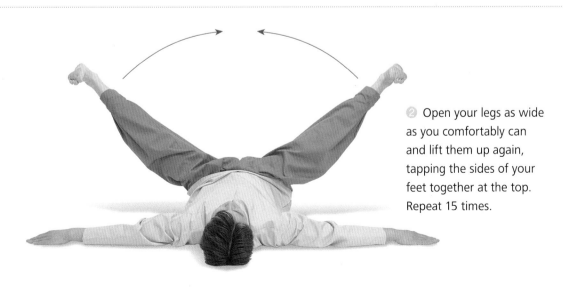

2. Open your legs as wide as you comfortably can and lift them up again, tapping the sides of your feet together at the top. Repeat 15 times.

STAMINA/ STRENGTHENING

Excessive stress and fatigue in a person's life can lead to a decrease in vital energy, or stamina. Lack of motivation and sexual desire can occur as well, as can sexual dysfunction, adversely affecting a person's intimate relationships and creating more stress.

Adherents of Eastern Medicine believe that the kidney controls the Jung energy, vital energy in the lower abdomen. The kidney and the liver are both vital organs—the kidney is responsible for filtering the blood, and the liver detoxifies the body. Both must be optimally functioning in order to develop and maintain stamina. The meridian exercises recommended in this chapter will enable optimal kidney and liver functioning and enhance overall vitality.

BICYCLE EXERCISE (P. 140)

BENEFITS Strengthens and stimulates lower extremities, muscles, and nerves around the perineal region and reproductive glands, thereby enabling heightened stamina.

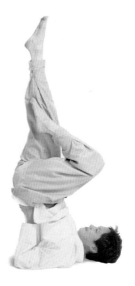

LEG LIFT (P. 226)

TIPS Avoid this exercise if you have hypertension or heart disease.

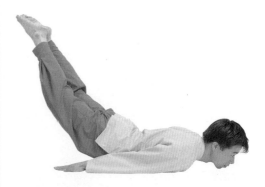

1. HOLDING TORSO LIFT

TIP If the floor is too hard, you can lie on a mat.

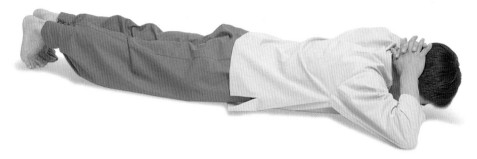

● Lie on your stomach with your legs extended and your toes flexed. Interlace your fingers behind your neck.

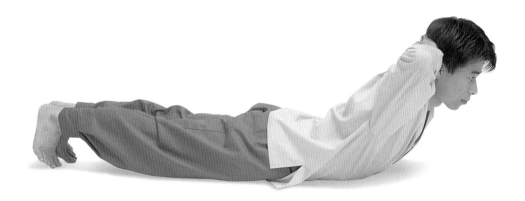

❷ Slowly lift your upper body off the floor and hold for as long as you comfortably can. Lower yourself to the floor. Repeat 10 times.

2. TIP TOE STRETCH

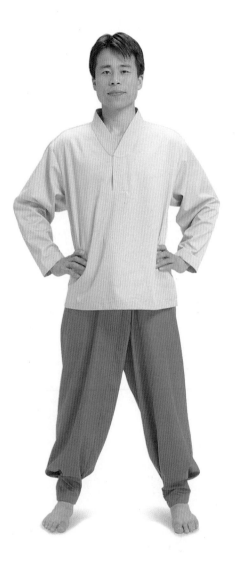

① Stand with your feet shoulder width apart and your hands on your waist. Relax your neck and shoulders.

② Inhale. Exhale slowly while bending from your hips to touch your palms to the floor with your fingers pointing toward one another.

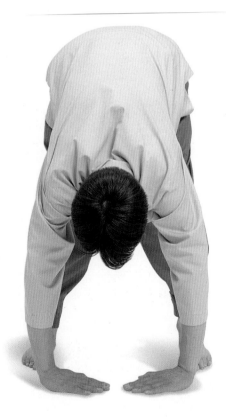

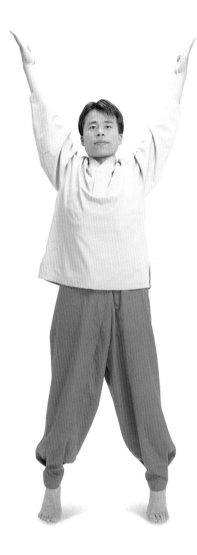

③ Inhale. Stand and raise both of your arms above your head, stretching with your palms toward the sky while simultaneously rising on your tiptoes. Exhale and slowly return to the original posture and repeat 3 times.

3. ANAL CONTRACTING EXERCISE FOR STAMINA/STRENGTHENING

BENEFITS Strengthens the reproductive system in men, assisting in remedying sexual dysfunction. Strengthens vaginal musculature in women.

① Sit in a half-lotus position or stand. Concentrate on lengthening the spine.

② Inhale as you distend your lower abdomen. Hold while contracting your anus.

③ Continue to hold for as long as you are comfortable. Exhale and relax the anus, but contract the abdominal muscles, pulling them toward your back. Perform this exercise for about 5 minutes. You can increase the time as you practice with consistency.

4. SIT-UP WITH FORWARD BEND

BENEFITS Strengthens the kidneys and waist area. Helps to correct sexual dysfunction.

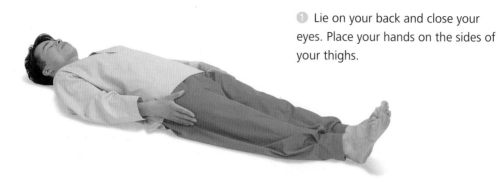

❶ Lie on your back and close your eyes. Place your hands on the sides of your thighs.

❷ Inhale through your nose. Hold the inhalation while gently lifting your torso. Rest your hands on the tops of your thighs.

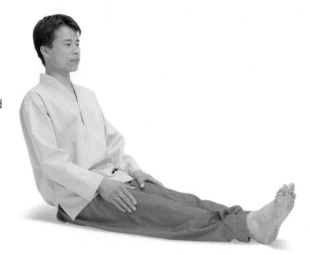

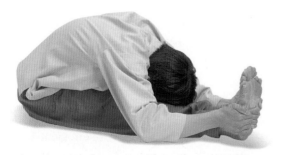

❸ Bend from your hips and slowly place both hands around the bottom of your feet. Hold for as long as comfortable. Exhale and return to STEP 1. Repeat 3 times.

5. THIGH TAPPING AND STRETCHING

BENEFITS Stimulates and strengthens the autonomic nervous system, particularly the reproductive glands. Strengthens stamina and improves sexual function.

TIPS Focus on the lower abdomen and relax the thighs and legs.

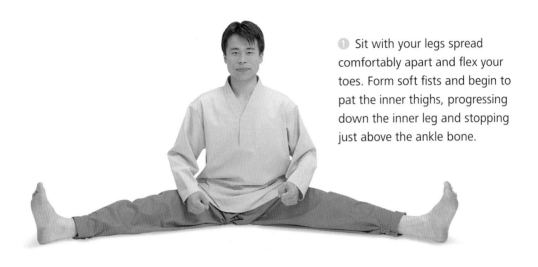

❶ Sit with your legs spread comfortably apart and flex your toes. Form soft fists and begin to pat the inner thighs, progressing down the inner leg and stopping just above the ankle bone.

❷ Place your hands palm down on the floor in front of you with your fingers pointing toward one another. Bounce your torso 10 times.

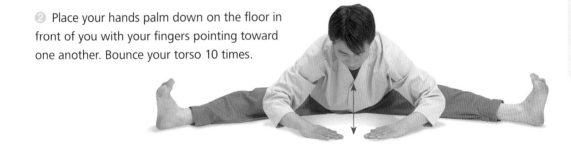

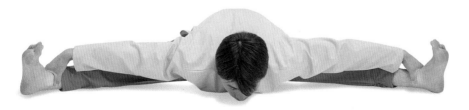

❸ Inhale. Place both hands on your ankles and bend from the hips, reaching your chin toward the floor. Return to a sitting position. Repeat 3 times.

6. LEG LIFT AND TWIST

BENEFITS Strengthens abdominal muscles to increase stamina and optimal sexual functioning. Prevents and alleviates lumbago. Prevents urological and reproductive system related disorders.

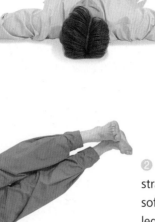

① Lie on your back with your arms extended at shoulder level. Lift both legs up to a 90-degree angle while keeping your feet flexed.

② Keeping your legs straight but your knees soft, slowly tilt both of your legs about 45 degrees to the left. Bring your legs back to the center.

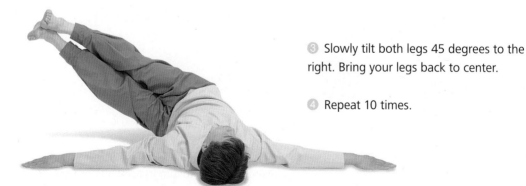

③ Slowly tilt both legs 45 degrees to the right. Bring your legs back to center.

④ Repeat 10 times.

7. TIPTOE BALANCE

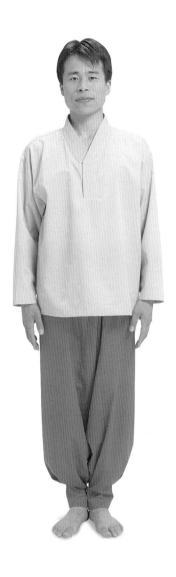 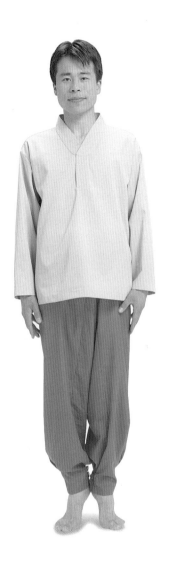

① Stand with your heels together and your toes about 3 inches apart. Relax your hands at your sides.

② Inhale. Keeping your heels together, lift them as much as you can. Hold your breath while simultaneously tightening the anal sphincter and the hip and leg muscles, and imagine pulling them toward your perineum. Focus on the perineal area.

③ Exhale, relax, and slowly lower your heels. Repeat 10 times.

EXERCISES FOR PREGNANCY

The process of birthing necessitates a tremendous surge of energy within a short period of time. During pregnancy, perform the recommended meridian exercises to accumulate vital energy and to maintain a healthy body, mind, and spirit in preparation for the challenge of labor. A healthy body can help to reduce pain during labor and decrease the chance of lasting physical effects caused by childbirth.

The meridian exercises recommended in this chapter are different from the other exercises in that they consider the growing fetus. Specifically, breathe naturally as opposed to holding your breath or intensifying breathing patterns. When assuming a breathing posture, do not raise your legs; rather, keep them on the floor. Close your eyes and relax as you concentrate and converse with your growing fetus.

FIRST TRIMESTER (0-3 MONTHS)

The first trimester requires you to be in touch with your body's natural rhythms instead of becoming unnecessarily distressed. Relaxing is extremely important for you and your developing baby.

TWISTING KNEE TOUCH (P. 196)

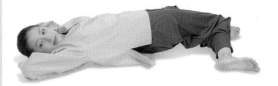

1. ANKLE JOINT EXERCISE

BENEFITS Opens up blockages to allow Ki energy and blood circulation to the lower extremities. Assists optimal reproductive system functioning during pregnancy.

① Sit or lie down with your hands behind you, fingers pointing away from you. Extend your legs straight out in front of you while maintaining soft knees. Slowly rotate your toes outward to form a circle. Feel the stretch in your ankles. Make at least 10 rotations in each direction.

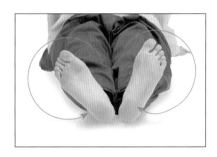

② Slowly alternate flexing and extending your feet. Focus on the muscles tightening and releasing. Flex and extend your feet 10 times.

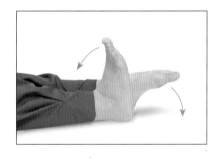

2. WHOLE BODY STRETCH

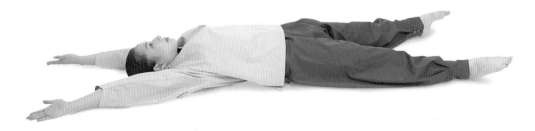

① Lie on your back with your legs extended, feet shoulder width apart. Slowly raise both hands and extend them on the floor above your head. Stretch your whole body, breathe out, and then release.

3. PUSH-UP WITH KNEE SUPPORT

BENEFITS Reduces excess pressure in the abdominal area while doing push-ups, which is especially important for pregnant women.

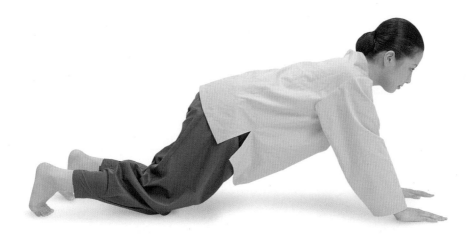

❶ Kneel with your toes flexed and place your hands on the floor in front of you, fingers facing forward.

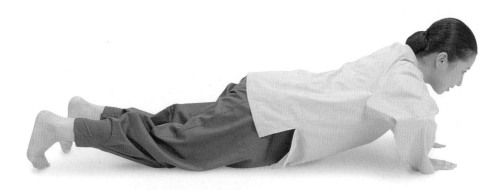

❷ Gently expand your chest, bend your elbows, and lower your upper body. Focus on keeping your upper legs and spine in a straight line. Extend your arms and return to the beginning position. Begin by performing 5 times. Increase repetitions as you practice regularly.

4. HIP LIFT

BENEFITS Strengthens and improves the elasticity of the pelvis while enhancing the digestive process.

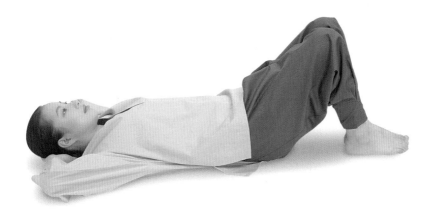

① Lie on your back with your knees bent and feet flat on the floor. Interlace your fingers behind your neck. Open your legs while bringing your heels close to your hips.

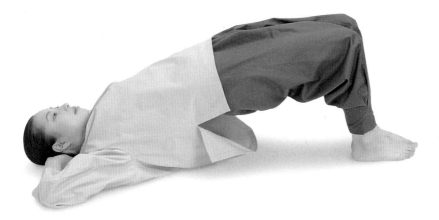

② Inhale. Raise your hips and waist while your shoulders and feet bear your weight. Touch your knees together and contract your pelvis.

③ Exhale. Lower your hips and waist. Repeat 3 times.

5. SIDE LEG LIFT

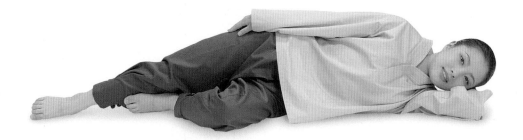

❶ Lie on your left side. Form
a pillow with your left arm
and rest your head on it
comfortably.

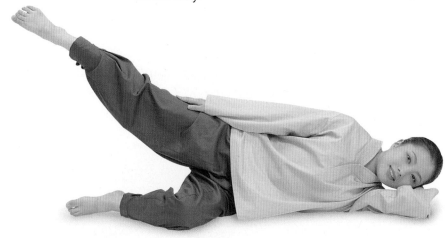

❷ Bend your left knee so your
left foot is in line with your right
knee. Place your right hand on
your right thigh. Inhale. Raise
your right leg up as far as you
comfortably can. Exhale and
bring it down. Repeat 10-20
times. Turn on your right side
and repeat leg lifting with your
left leg.

6. CIRCULATION SHAKE

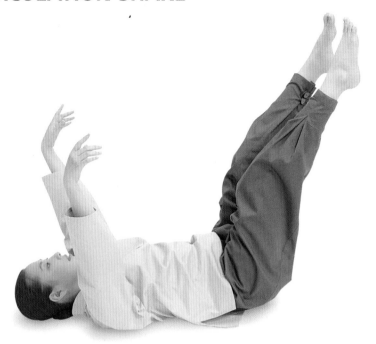

❶ Lie on your back. Raise your arms and legs and shake gently for 3 minutes.

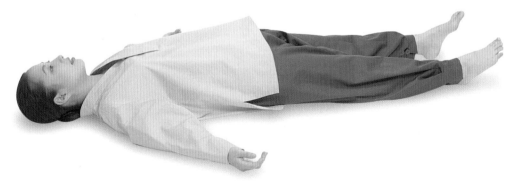

❷ Drop your arms and legs. Relax your body.

SECOND TRIMESTER (4-6 MONTHS)

During the second trimester, the fetus is settled in the uterus, thereby decreasing the liability to the mother and fetus. Exercise levels can be increased with more comfort and safety, though you should still do so with caution and with the approval of your labor and delivery consultant. The meridian exercises recommended in this section condition the body to be strong during the ensuing months of pregnancy and labor.

1. SHOULDER SHRUGGING

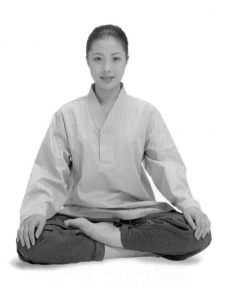
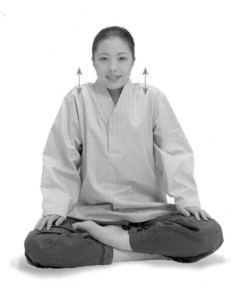

❶ Sit in a half-lotus position. Relax your shoulders. Inhale and raise your shoulders toward your ears. Exhale and drop your shoulders. Repeat 3-5 times.

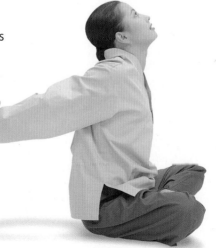

❷ Interlace your fingers behind your back and open your chest. Inhale and tilt your head back for about 5 seconds. Exhale and return to the beginning posture.

2. SITTING SIDE BEND

BENEFITS Promotes elasticity, flexibility, and mobility in the waist and sides of torso while preventing and easing discomfort of the lower back.

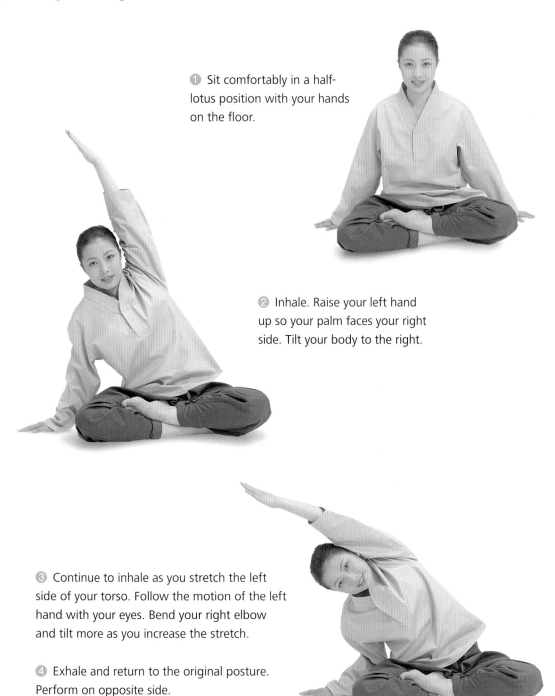

❶ Sit comfortably in a half-lotus position with your hands on the floor.

❷ Inhale. Raise your left hand up so your palm faces your right side. Tilt your body to the right.

❸ Continue to inhale as you stretch the left side of your torso. Follow the motion of the left hand with your eyes. Bend your right elbow and tilt more as you increase the stretch.

❹ Exhale and return to the original posture. Perform on opposite side.

3. BUTTERFLY FLAPPING

TIPS Stimulates the Jang-gang (Du 1) acupressure point, located in the region of the coccyx and perineum. Sit on a blanket or mat to provide more cushioning for you and your fetus. Flap your legs gently, without causing strain.

EXERCISES FOR PREGNANCY

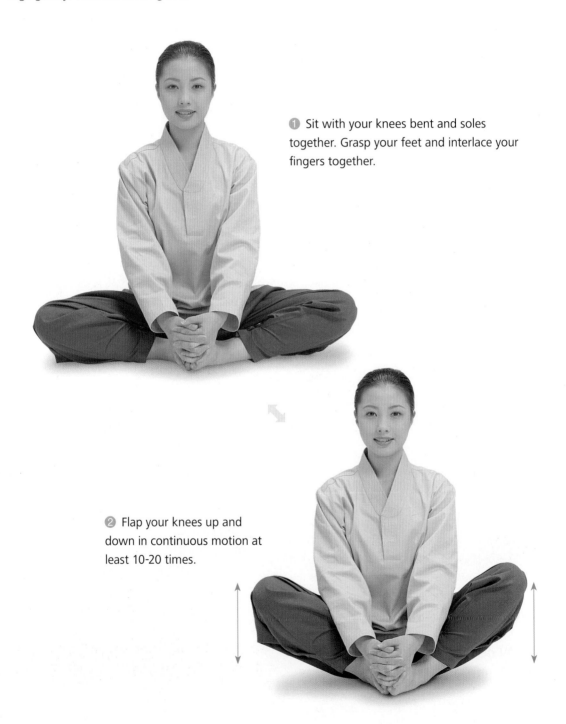

❶ Sit with your knees bent and soles together. Grasp your feet and interlace your fingers together.

❷ Flap your knees up and down in continuous motion at least 10-20 times.

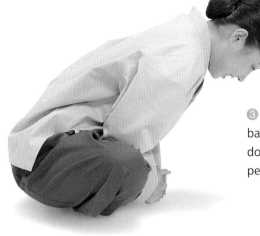

❸ Lean forward with your upper body. Rock back and forth while lifting your hips up and down to stimulate the Jang-gang point and perineum.

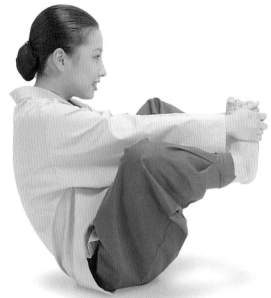

❹ Continue to grasp your feet with your hands and raise them to chest level, tilting your upper body backward to keep your balance. Hold for as long as you comfortably can.

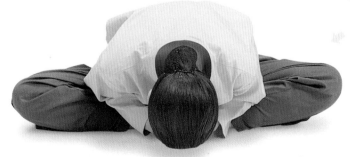

❺ Rest your feet on the floor again and pull them toward your body. Gently and slowly lower your upper body and your head toward your feet as much as you can without straining. Hold and release. Repeat 2 more times.

4. CAT STRETCH

BENEFITS Helps uterus to accommodate increasing size and necessary mobility for the developing fetus.

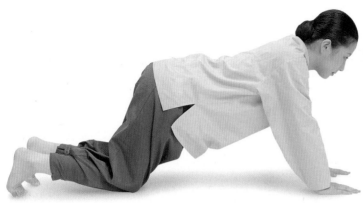

① Kneel with your toes flexed and your hands on the floor below your shoulders.

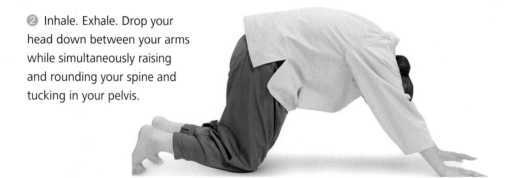

② Inhale. Exhale. Drop your head down between your arms while simultaneously raising and rounding your spine and tucking in your pelvis.

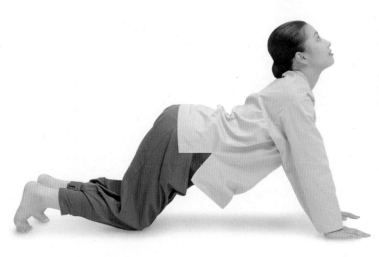

③ Inhale. Exhale and raise your head to look toward the sky. Simultaneously arch your spine into a lion posture.

④ Inhale. Return to STEP 1. Repeat 3-5 times.

5. SITTING SIDE BEND VARIATION

BENEFITS Realigns the pelvis. Enhances Ki energy and blood circulation as it warms the lower abdomen.

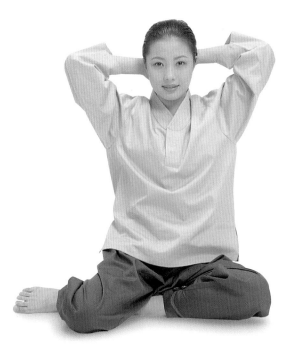

❶ Sit with your knees bent, your right foot to the side near your right hip and your left foot resting beneath your right thigh. Interlace your fingers behind your head.

❷ Inhale. Slowly bend toward the right.

❸ Exhale and return to center. Inhale and bend to the left, and exhale again to the center. Repeat in each direction one more time.

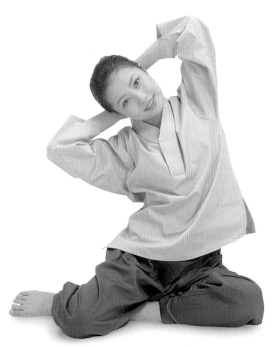

LAST TRIMESTER (7 MONTHS UNTIL BIRTH)

During the last trimester, anxiety can mount as you anticipate the birth of the baby. It is helpful to apply measures that will boost your mind, body, and spirit toward optimal relaxation. Listening to peaceful music and doing other activities that you associate with a relaxed state of mind are helpful. Furthermore, with the increased weight gain during this trimester, you might become more sedentary and fatigued, leading to less exercise and weakening muscles. The recommended exercises in this section help to keep you active while the abdominal breathing aids in achieving relaxation.

1. PIGEON TOE SQUATS

BENEFITS Strengthens thigh muscles, external genital region, and anal sphincter muscles. Facilitates release of muscular tension to ease the baby's passage through the birth canal and decrease the mother's pain during labor.

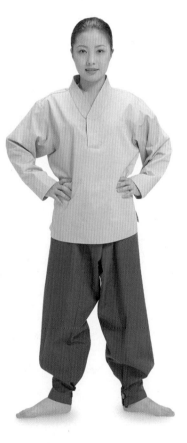

❶ Stand with your hands on your waist, feet shoulder width apart, and your toes pointing outward.

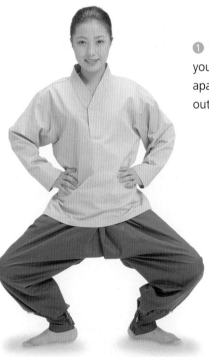

❷ Inhale. Bend your knees to a comfortable level. Exhale and stand up. Repeat 12 times.

2. KNEELING ARCH

BENEFITS Strengthens and realigns the spine, waist, and legs to decrease pain during delivery.

TIP If surface is too hard for kneeling, perform this exercise on a mat.

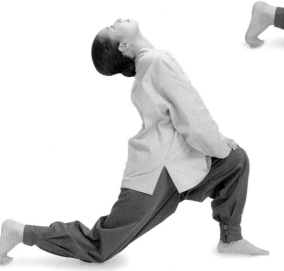

❶ Kneel on your right knee with the toes of your right foot flexed. Place your left foot in front of you with your knee bent 90 degrees.

❷ Place your hands on your left knee. Slowly arch your back and head backward as you concentrate on opening the chest. Hold and release. Repeat for the opposite side.

STRADDLE STRETCH (P. 274)

TIP Bend slowly and gently so as not to place undue pressure on your abdomen.

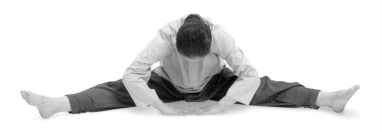

Exercises for Women   *255*

3. LEG LIFT

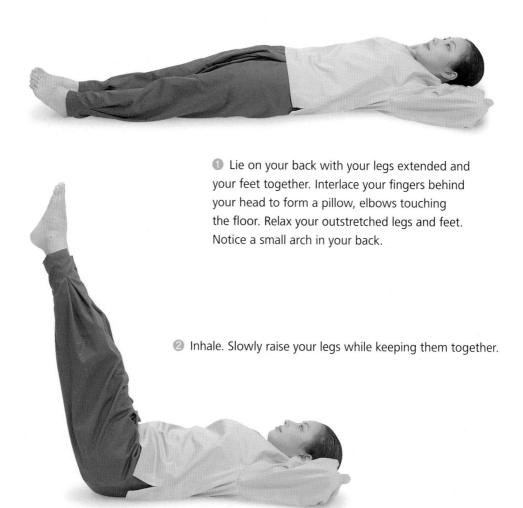

❶ Lie on your back with your legs extended and your feet together. Interlace your fingers behind your head to form a pillow, elbows touching the floor. Relax your outstretched legs and feet. Notice a small arch in your back.

❷ Inhale. Slowly raise your legs while keeping them together.

❸ Exhale. Slowly lower your legs but do not touch the floor. Repeat 5 times.

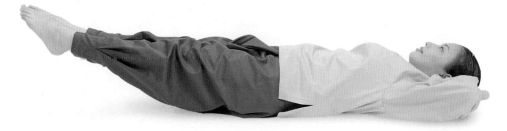

4. WAIST LIFT

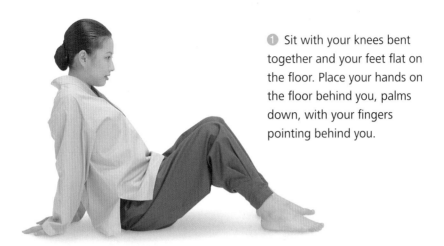

① Sit with your knees bent together and your feet flat on the floor. Place your hands on the floor behind you, palms down, with your fingers pointing behind you.

② Inhale. Lift your waist up to form a bridge. Tilt your head back with your face to the sky.

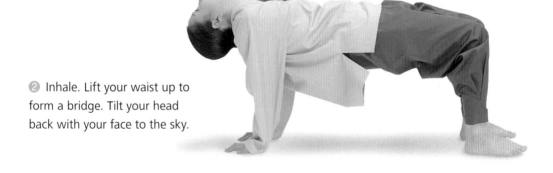

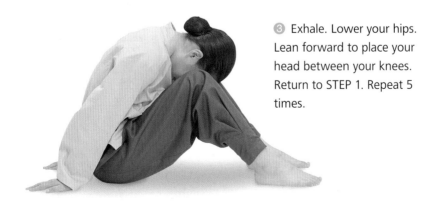

③ Exhale. Lower your hips. Lean forward to place your head between your knees. Return to STEP 1. Repeat 5 times.

5. BABY POSTURE

TIP Breathe naturally without forcing your abdomen in and out.

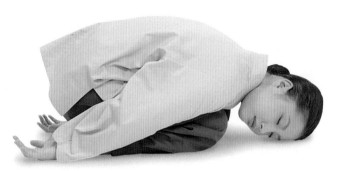

❶ Kneel on the floor with your feet relaxed and toes pointing behind you. Allow your knees to separate at a comfortable angle, and lean your upper body forward until your head rests on the floor, facing whichever direction is most comfortable. Rest your arms comfortably at your sides with your palms facing up. Hold for as long as is comfortable.

6. RESTING WITH FEET ELEVATED AGAINST THE WALL

BENEFITS Relieves fatigue in the lower back, common in pregnant women and people who stand for long periods of time.

❶ Lie on your back with your hips near a wall and extend your arms to your sides at shoulder level. Raise your legs so your feet rest shoulder width apart on the wall. Breathe normally and comfortably.

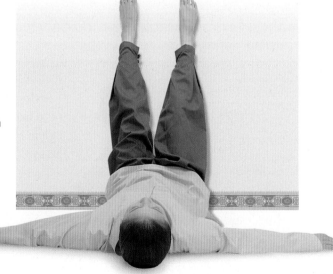

7. TIGHTENING FISTS AND STRETCHING WITH PRAYER HANDS

TIPS When first performing this exercise, repeat slowly 10 times. As you progress in your practice, you can increase to 30 times at a faster pace.

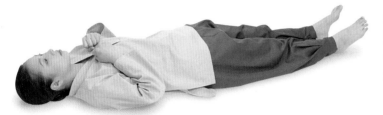

❶ Lie on your back with your legs extended. Form soft fists with both of your hands and rest them on your chest.

❷ Flex your hands to form strong fists. Open and close forcefully 15 times.

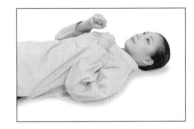

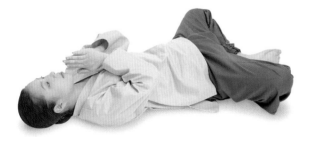

❸ Place your hands in a prayer position and bend your knees to bring the soles of your feet together.

❹ Inhale. Exhale. Place your arms over your head with your palms together and feet relaxed.

❺ Inhale. Return to STEP 3 and repeat. Repeat 2 more times.

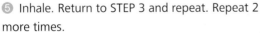

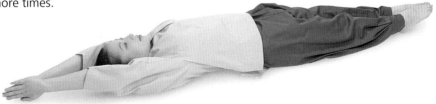

POSTPARTUM RECOVERY

Immediately following birth, your bones are soft and your joints and organs need to be realigned. Two or three days of full rest are needed to begin the healing process. To prevent hemorrhaging, only light activity is recommended during the initial six-week postpartum time period.

The recommended meridian exercises in this section are particularly beneficial to the postpartum woman, as they begin with lying postures and progress to standing postures to support your recovery. Proceed with caution to avoid straining your joints and muscles during your exercise movements. Practice these exercises for about two months and consult with your labor and delivery adviser before proceeding to standing postures.

ANKLE JOINT EXERCISE
(P. 243)

BENEFITS Stimulates the Urinary Bladder Meridian and strengthens the reproductive system. Enhances stomach and liver function.

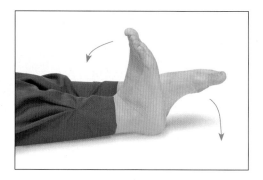

TIGHTENING FISTS
(P. 259)

BENEFITS Helps blood circulation and decreases swelling in arms and hands.

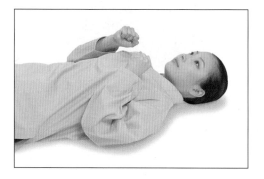

1. WAIST TWIST

BENEFITS Realigns the pelvis and relaxes the waist area.

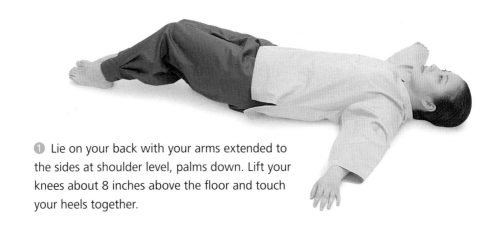

① Lie on your back with your arms extended to the sides at shoulder level, palms down. Lift your knees about 8 inches above the floor and touch your heels together.

② Gently rock your knees to the right side, allowing your body to move. Simultaneously turn your head to the left. Repeat to the other side and continue in a rocking motion. Repeat this motion for each direction several times.

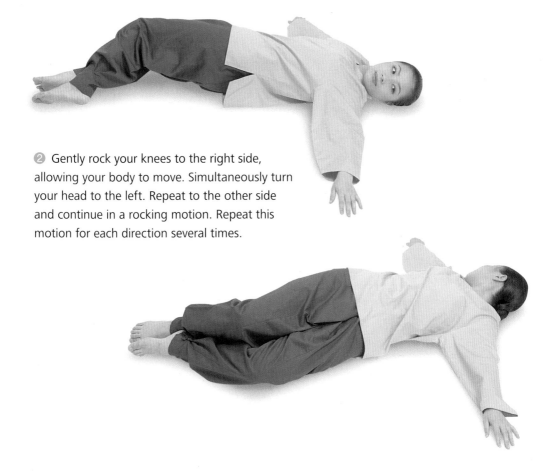

2. PELVIC TWIST

TIP Perform each motion very slowly.

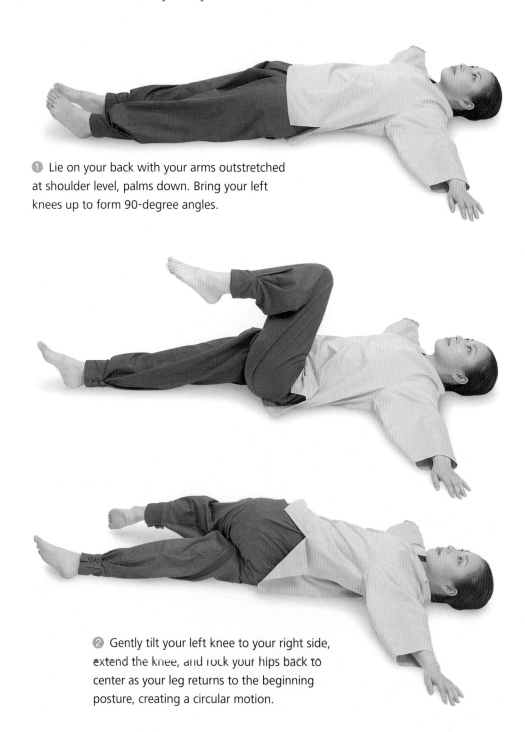

❶ Lie on your back with your arms outstretched at shoulder level, palms down. Bring your left knees up to form 90-degree angles.

❷ Gently tilt your left knee to your right side, extend the knee, and rock your hips back to center as your leg returns to the beginning posture, creating a circular motion.

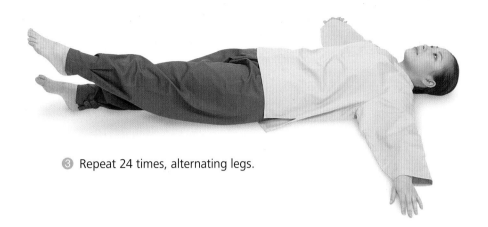

③ Repeat 24 times, alternating legs.

3. ABDOMINAL BREATHING

BENEFITS Replenishes Ki energy expended at the time of the birth. Revitalizes the body's harmonious symmetry and realigns bones and organs.

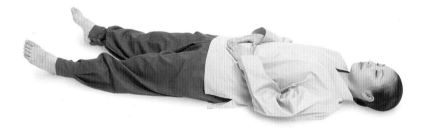

❶ Lie on your back with your legs extended and feet shoulder width apart. Place your hands on your Dahn-jon, forming a triangle with your thumbs and fingers. Focus on your lower abdomen. Perform abdominal breathing comfortably for 2-3 minutes.

❷ Turn onto your stomach with your head to one side with your hands resting at your sides. Continue abdominal breathing.

LEUKORRHEA

Leukorrhea, or discharge from the vagina, is experienced by many women. It is accompanied by a chill around the waist, lower abdomen, and knees. It can, if left untreated, cause irregular menstruation and infertility. It results from the malfunction of blood circulation in the lower extremities, and the imbalance of sexual hormones due to birth, miscarriage, or birth control medicines and devices. Certain foods, such as ginger root, potatoes, onions, and radishes, can be helpful to increase body warmth, and it is best to avoid artificial seasonings and sugar.

The recommended exercises in this section assist you in enhancing the depth of your abdominal breathing and expelling coldness from your body. People with hypertension should refrain from breathing with this intensity and carry out abdominal breathing as regularly prescribed. Initially, you may experience a deeper sensation of chills and body aches, but within two to three months, you should notice an increase in your body temperature and a decrease of symptoms related to leukorrhea.

WHOLE BODY PATTING (P. 20)

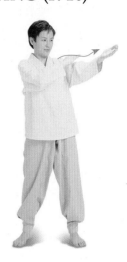

CIRCULATION EXERCISE (P. 24)

BENEFITS Helps blood circulation and decreases swelling in hands and arms.

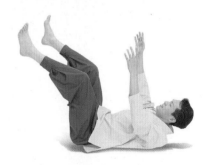

SITTING FORWARD BEND (P. 50)

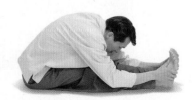

BRIDGE POSTURE (P. 199)

BENEFITS Flexes the whole body, particularly the neck, hips, waist, and shoulders. Releases tension. Controls Yin-Yang Ki energy flow, thereby harmonizing the balance in the body.

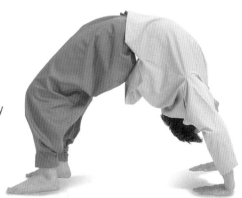

1. TAILBONE TAPPING

BENEFITS Releases Ki energy blockage in the tailbone area, which then alleviates coldness, leukorrhea, and some sexual dysfunctions.

❶ Sit with your legs crossed and place the palm of your hand on the tailbone area. Gently pat the area where the acupressure points are located for about one minute.

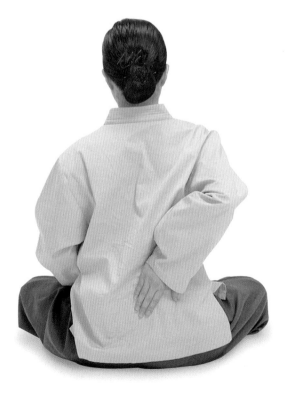

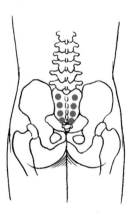

Eight acupressure points around the tailbone.

2. PUSHING PALM BODY TWIST

TIPS When you perform these movements, focus on keeping your chest open and elongating the spine.

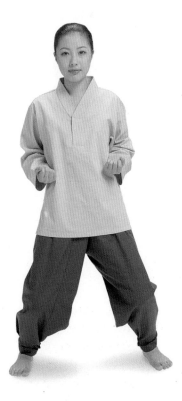

❶ Stand with your knees slightly bent and your feet a little more than shoulder width apart. Hold your hands palm up at your sides and close them into fists.

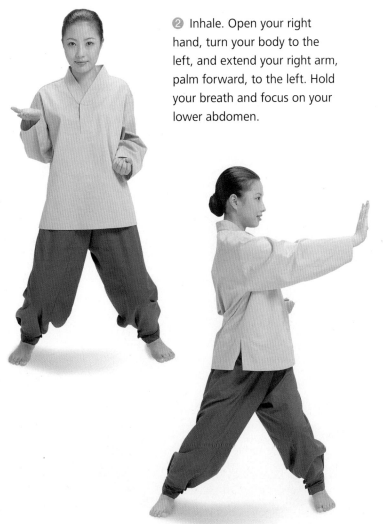

❷ Inhale. Open your right hand, turn your body to the left, and extend your right arm, palm forward, to the left. Hold your breath and focus on your lower abdomen.

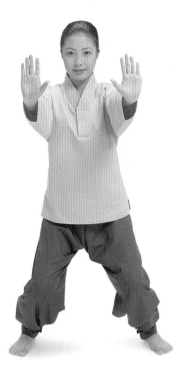

❸ Exhale. Return to the original position. Inhale, open your left hand, and turn your body to the right, pushing your palm out to the right side. Hold your breath and return to center.

❹ Inhale. Open your hands and flex your wrists so your fingers point toward the floor. Slowly raise your hands toward your shoulders. Then bend your knees while you rotate your fingers to point upward and push the centers of your palms straight out in front, palms facing away. Exhale and return to center.

3. CROSSED BOW POSTURE

BENEFITS Releases stagnant blood and Ki energy from abdominal area. Strengthens spine. Helps to alleviate leukorrhea and constipation.

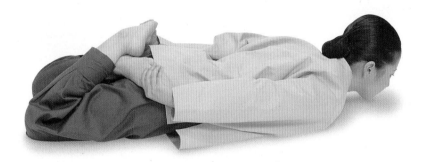

❶ Lie on your stomach. Bend your knees and cross your feet.

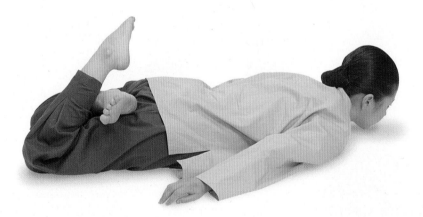

❷ Hold your feet with both of your hands.

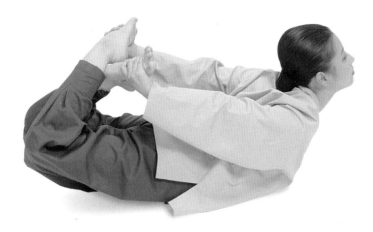

❸ Gently pull your feet and lift your upper torso and head to form an arch in your back. Hold this position for 30 seconds.

❹ Switch the crossing position of your feet and repeat 4 times on each side.

4. TOE WIGGLE LEG LIFT

BENEFITS Helps to bring relief from insomnia, anxiety, headache, low stamina, and the cold sensation associated with leukorrhea by activating the many meridians located in the feet which are connected to body functions.

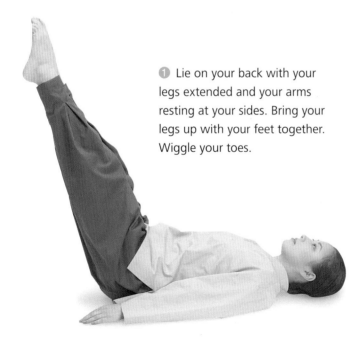

❶ Lie on your back with your legs extended and your arms resting at your sides. Bring your legs up with your feet together. Wiggle your toes.

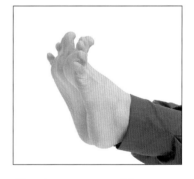

❷ Rub your toes and feet together. Practice spreading your toes apart as much as possible without touching them with your hands. Spread your toes apart for several seconds and then release. Repeat several times.

5. LEG LIFT VARIATION

❶ Lie on your back with your legs extended, feet together, and your arms resting at your sides. Inhale. Raise your right leg to a 90-degree angle. Keep your knee soft but not bent. Flex your ankle and notice the tightness in the thigh and lower abdomen.

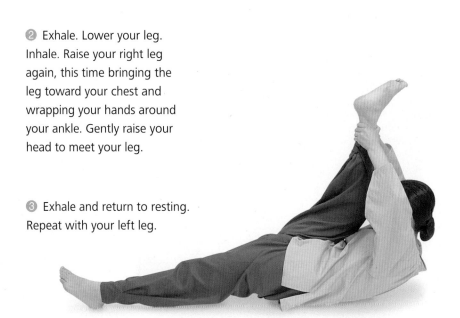

❷ Exhale. Lower your leg. Inhale. Raise your right leg again, this time bringing the leg toward your chest and wrapping your hands around your ankle. Gently raise your head to meet your leg.

❸ Exhale and return to resting. Repeat with your left leg.

6. KNEELING BACK BEND

TIPS Do not overexert yourself with this exercise if you have back pain. Do not perform this exercise if you have hypertension.

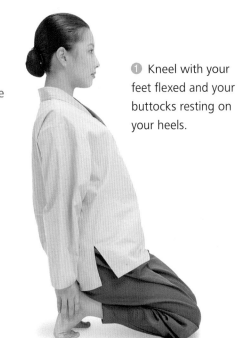

❶ Kneel with your feet flexed and your buttocks resting on your heels.

❷ Grasp your ankles with your hands. Inhale and raise your waist while tilting your head back. Simultaneously contract your anus and open your chest.

❸ Return to original posture as you exhale.

❹ Inhale and repeat STEP 2.

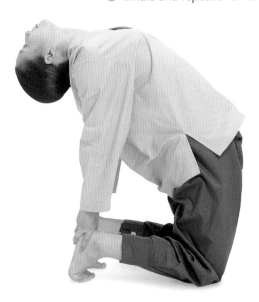

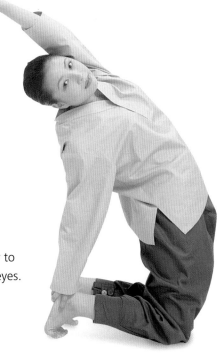

❺ Hold your breath. Raise your left arm to touch your left ear and tilt your upper body to the right. Follow your fingertips with your eyes. Return to STEP 1 as you exhale.

❻ Switch arms and repeat.

MENSTRUAL DISORDERS

Adherents of Eastern Medicine believe that cramps accompanying menstruation are the result of coldness and stagnant blood in the area of the pelvis. This weakens the uterus, ovaries, and muscles near the pelvis, causing fatigue, headache, anxiety, hypersensitivity, abdominal cramps, and excessive menstruation. You might even experience spasms caused by the intestines twisting. Menstrual cramping can also occur if there is blockage in the Conception Vessel (Immaek), low Ki energy in the kidney, or overall body fragility.

The recommended meridian exercises benefit women who suffer from menstrual pain, irregular menstruation, or diseases that affect the uterus. In addition to performing the recommended exercises, it can be helpful to lie on your stomach on a warm surface or heating pad to dissipate the cramping and facilitate a sense of serenity. Also, rub your hands together until they are warm and place them on your abdomen, rubbing clockwise to alleviate the pain. And lastly, avoid excessive meridian exercises during menstruation.

LYING HIP BOUNCE (P. 98)

BENEFITS Opens the Myung-moon acupressure point. Enhances essential organ functions and helps to reduce lower back pain.

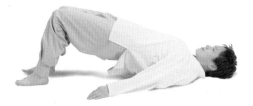

FORWARD BUTTERFLY BEND (P. 123)

BENEFITS Helps to circulate Ki energy to the lower abdomen, relieving menstrual cramps and regulating menstruation. Calms the mind and enhances skin radiance.

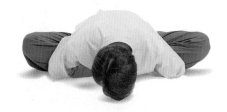

LEG LIFT (P. 226)

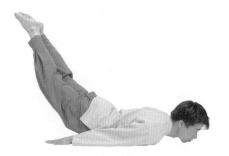

1. REPRODUCTIVE ACUPRESSURE

BENEFITS Helps to relieve knee pain, uterine bleeding, and excessive bleeding during menstruation. Helps to heal reproductive problems in both women and men.

TIP If you are pregnant, do not press too hard on the Sp 6 points.

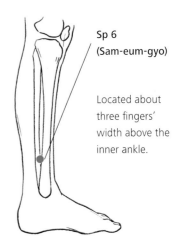

Sp 6
(Sam-eum-gyo)

Located about three fingers' width above the inner ankle.

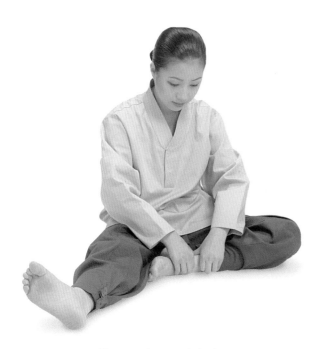

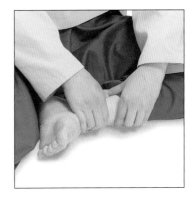

❶ Sit with your right leg extended and your left knee bent, the sole of your left foot against your right knee. With both thumbs, press on the Sp 6 acupressure point.

❷ Inhale. Continue to press your Sp 6 points. Apply upper body weight as you press on this acupressure point.

❸ Exhale. Release your thumbs.

2. STRADDLE STRETCH

BENEFITS Assists in eliminating fat from the thighs and the abdominal area—particularly beneficial in alleviating symptoms of diabetes and menstrual cramping. Helps to realign the lumbar and sacral areas of the spine.

❶ From a sitting posture, open your legs as far apart as comfortable. Place both of your hands on the floor, palms down and elbows bent. Bounce lightly from the hips and maintain your focus on your thighs.

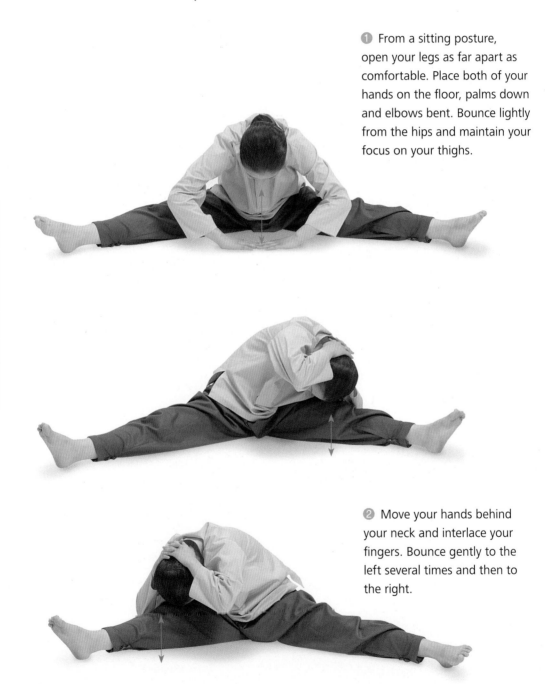

❷ Move your hands behind your neck and interlace your fingers. Bounce gently to the left several times and then to the right.

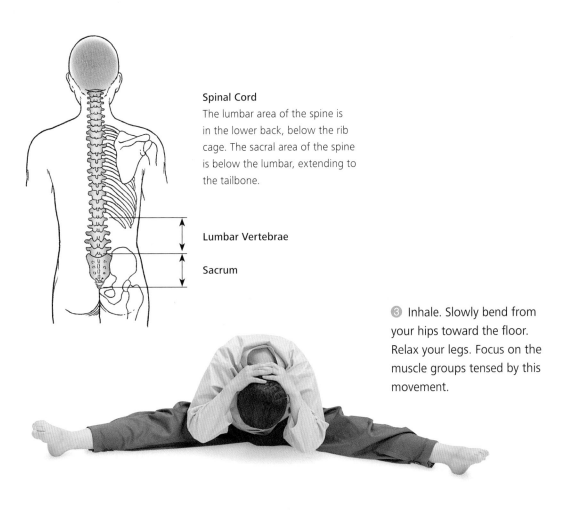

Spinal Cord
The lumbar area of the spine is in the lower back, below the rib cage. The sacral area of the spine is below the lumbar, extending to the tailbone.

Lumbar Vertebrae

Sacrum

❸ Inhale. Slowly bend from your hips toward the floor. Relax your legs. Focus on the muscle groups tensed by this movement.

KIDNEY ACUPRESSURE (P. 224)

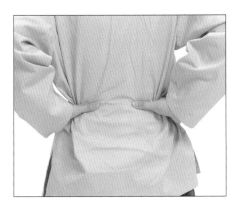

BENEFITS Helps to relieve lumbago pain. Also improves kidney function and treats reproductive disorders in men and women.

3. PRAYER BEND

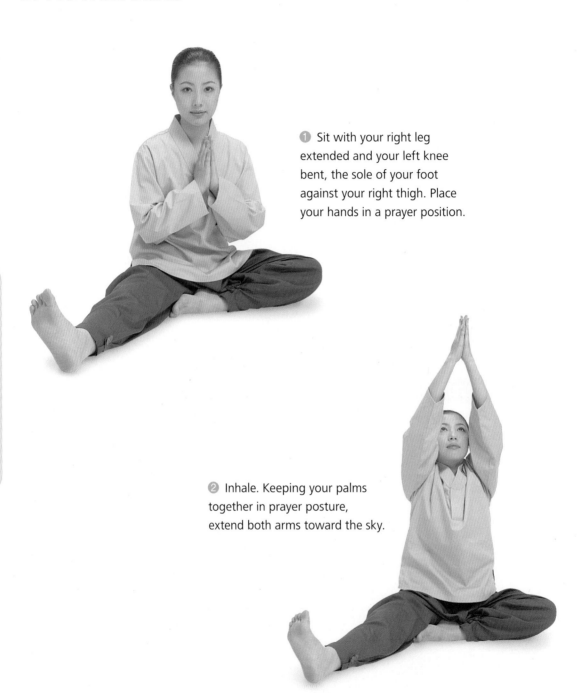

❶ Sit with your right leg extended and your left knee bent, the sole of your foot against your right thigh. Place your hands in a prayer position.

❷ Inhale. Keeping your palms together in prayer posture, extend both arms toward the sky.

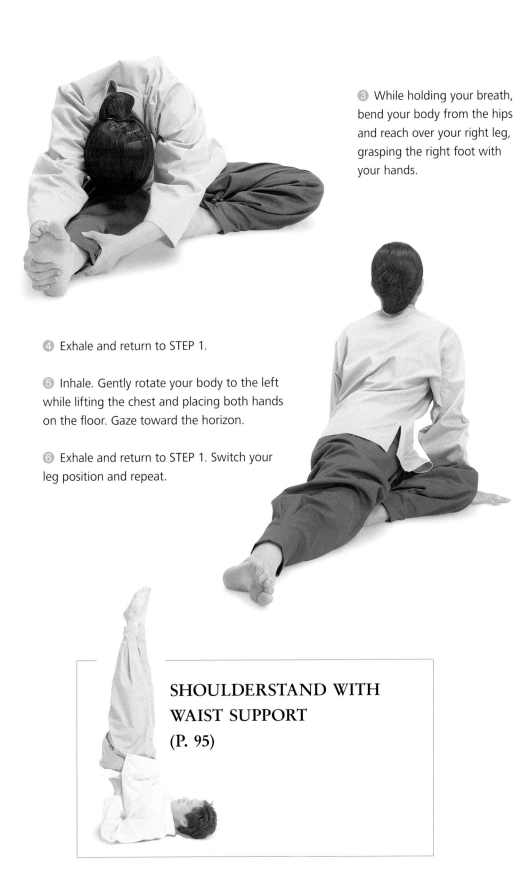

③ While holding your breath, bend your body from the hips and reach over your right leg, grasping the right foot with your hands.

④ Exhale and return to STEP 1.

⑤ Inhale. Gently rotate your body to the left while lifting the chest and placing both hands on the floor. Gaze toward the horizon.

⑥ Exhale and return to STEP 1. Switch your leg position and repeat.

SHOULDERSTAND WITH WAIST SUPPORT (P. 95)

OBESITY

Obesity results from the accumulation of excessive amounts of fat within the body. It can increase your risk of contracting a multitude of diseases and conditions, including diabetes, stroke, heart disease, certain types of cancer, respiratory disorders, gall stones, sleep apnea, and high blood pressure.

The meridian exercises recommended in this section facilitate the shedding of excess fat from the body. Intestinal function is enhanced as the blood and Ki energy circulation of the digestive system are stimulated. This revitalizes brain cells and the metabolic system, igniting fat-burning activity and normalizing hormone secretions. Consistent practice of these exercises facilitates appetite control as well. Through the synthesis of these changes, you can notice an improvement in well-being and a more positive attitude toward life.

WHOLE BODY PATTING (P. 20)

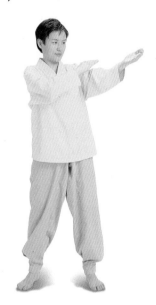

ABDOMINAL CLAPPING (P. 25)

BENEFITS Relieves gas accumulation in the intestines and eliminates excess fat from the lower abdomen.

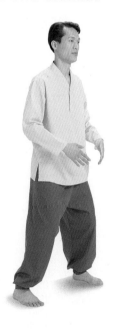

INTESTINE EXERCISE
(P. 26)

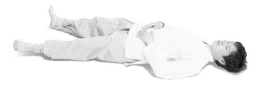

BICYCLE EXERCISE
(P. 140)

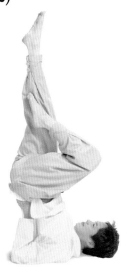

PIGEON TOE SQUATS
(P. 254)

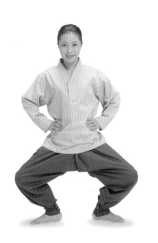

PULLING KNEES TO CHEST
(P. 105)

BENEFITS Realigns pelvis and removes gas from the intestines. Helps to strengthen and lift the buttocks.

ARM TWIST (P. 154)

BENEFITS Enhances flexibility in the wrists, arms, and shoulder blades. Breaks down the fats of the arm muscle to promote leanness. Helps to relieve fatigue and numbness as well as tingling in the arms.

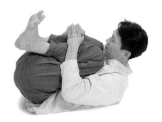

LEG LIFT VARIATION
(P. 270)

BENEFITS Relieves accumulation of stagnant blood and toxins in the lower extremities and eliminates fat accumulation from the abdomen and thigh areas.

1. SIDE BEND

BENEFITS Shapes waist, legs, and sides. Helps to reduce fat around the shoulders and under the arms.

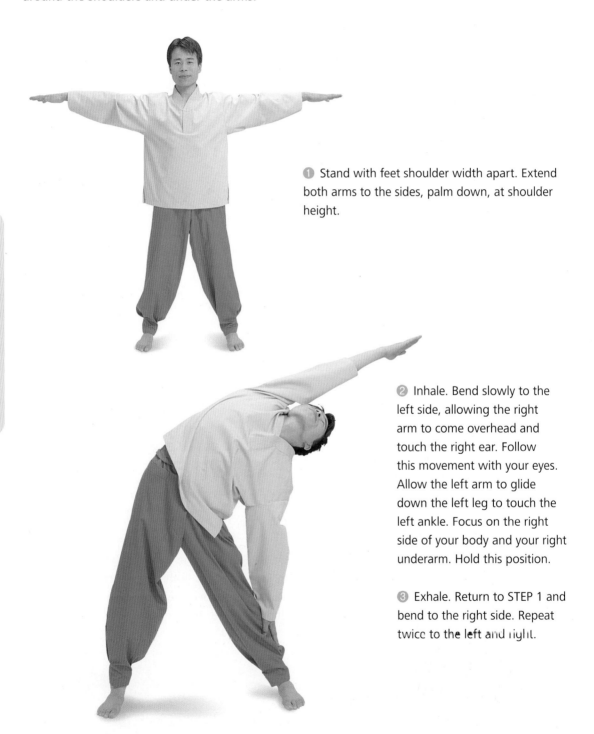

① Stand with feet shoulder width apart. Extend both arms to the sides, palm down, at shoulder height.

② Inhale. Bend slowly to the left side, allowing the right arm to come overhead and touch the right ear. Follow this movement with your eyes. Allow the left arm to glide down the left leg to touch the left ankle. Focus on the right side of your body and your right underarm. Hold this position.

③ Exhale. Return to STEP 1 and bend to the right side. Repeat twice to the left and right.

2. GROIN STRETCH

BENEFITS Strengthens thighs and buttocks while helping to shape the legs and hips.

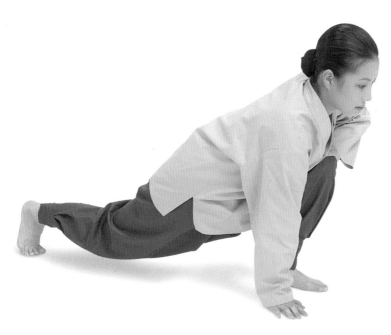

❶ Stand with your left leg in front of your right. With your left hand on your left knee for support, bend your left knee and lean forward to place your right hand on the floor, parallel to the left foot. Stretch your right leg back, toes flexed.

❷ Lower your hips and look toward the horizon while you bounce up and down gently several times. Then lower your hips farther while holding this position for as long as you comfortably can.

❸ Repeat with the opposite leg.

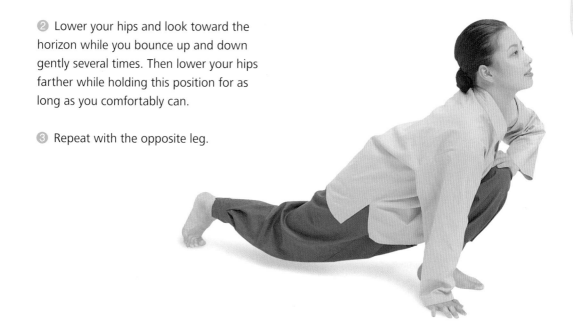

3. HALF-MOON STRADDLE

BENEFITS Enhances liver and digestive system function. Flexes and shapes the waist and legs. Stimulates the reproductive system, thereby increasing stamina.

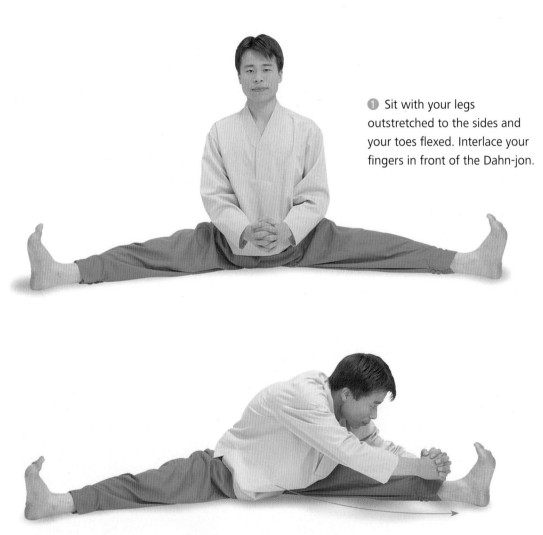

❶ Sit with your legs outstretched to the sides and your toes flexed. Interlace your fingers in front of the Dahn-jon.

❷ Slowly move your body with a circular motion toward the left toes and follow this movement with your eyes.

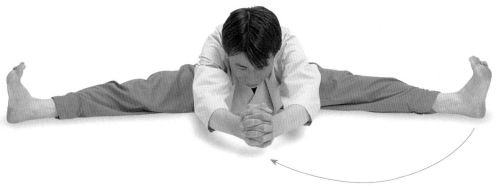

❸ Expand the circular motion
and slowly bring your body
to the center, parallel to your
Dahn-jon.

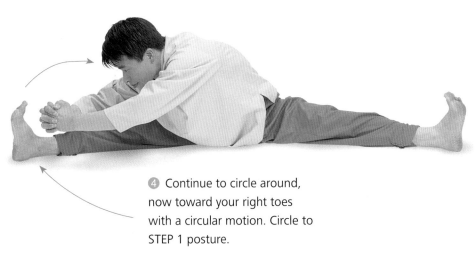

❹ Continue to circle around,
now toward your right toes
with a circular motion. Circle to
STEP 1 posture.

❺ Repeat the motion 3 times,
alternating directions.

4. SUPERMAN POSTURE VARIATION

BENEFITS Helps to shape the back and waist.

TIPS Perform this exercise as soon as you awaken in the morning. When you lift your arms and legs, proceed very slowly and with only a few repetitions, not exceeding 10 times in the beginning.

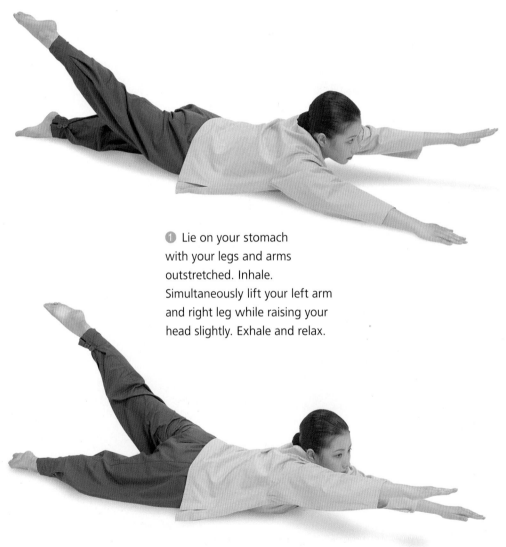

❶ Lie on your stomach with your legs and arms outstretched. Inhale. Simultaneously lift your left arm and right leg while raising your head slightly. Exhale and relax.

❷ Inhale and raise your right arm and left leg while raising your head slightly. Repeat the motion 5 times.

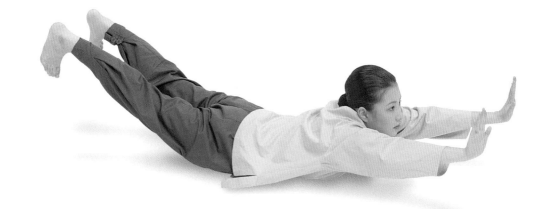

③ Inhale. Simultaneously lift both arms and legs very gently with only your Dahn-jon touching the floor.

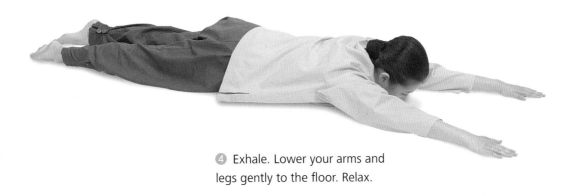

④ Exhale. Lower your arms and legs gently to the floor. Relax.

5. HEAD ROTATION

BENEFITS Releases tension from the muscles in the neck and helps to reshape them. Enhances the quality of the voice.

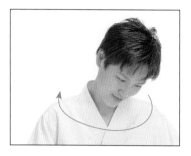

❶ Stand, or sit in a half-lotus position. Begin very slowly to rotate your head by tilting it first to the right, and then to the back, to the left, and then forward, in a 360-degree rotation. Then repeat to the other side.

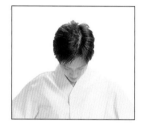 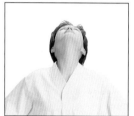 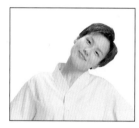 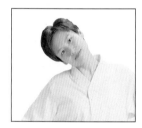

❷ Slowly move your head toward your chest and back and then toward the right shoulder and the left shoulder.

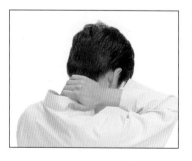 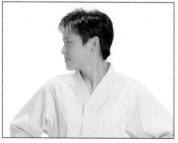

❸ Inhale. Sit still. Turn your head to the left very slowly. Hold it for a few seconds and then exhale to the center. Repeat on the right side. Repeat the sequence 5 times.

❹ Massage the back of your neck with your right hand and then with your left hand.

6. NECK LIFT

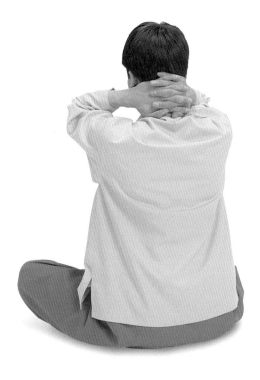

❶ Interlace your fingers behind your neck.

❷ Gently tilt your head back while lifting your neck. Slowly release. Repeat 4-5 times.

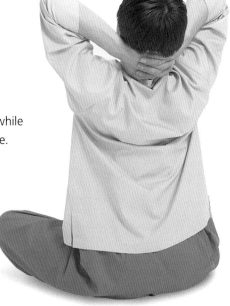

7. SIT-UP VARIATION

BENEFITS Reshapes abdominal muscles.

TIPS It is important to practice this exercise consistently to achieve maximum benefit. When you lift your upper body, proceed cautiously, using your entire upper body. Make certain that you do not bounce or exert undue effort with your shoulders. Maintain focus on your abdominal muscles to assist you while lifting. If the recommended 30 repetitions are too difficult, then begin with only a few repetitions and increase as you consistently practice.

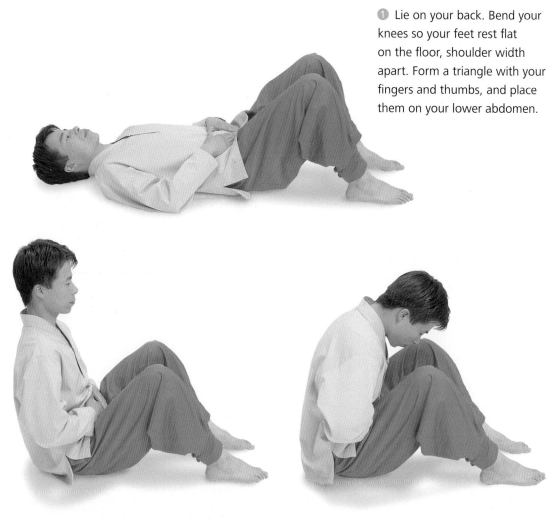

❶ Lie on your back. Bend your knees so your feet rest flat on the floor, shoulder width apart. Form a triangle with your fingers and thumbs, and place them on your lower abdomen.

❷ Focus on your lower abdomen. Slowly lift your upper body. Repeat 30 times.

8. ANKLE JOINT EXERCISE

BENEFITS Effects shapely appearance of the ankles.

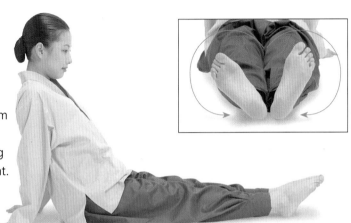

❶ Sit with your legs comfortably outstretched in front of you. Place your hands on the floor behind you with your fingers pointing away from you body. Slowly rotate your ankles 360 degrees, alternating the direction of your movement.

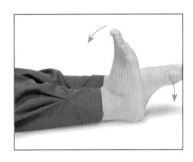

❷ Point the toes of one foot while simultaneously flexing the other foot. Switch and repeat several times.

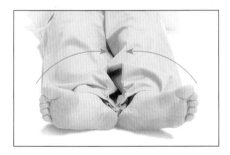

❸ Keep your heels touching while you drop your little toes to the floor and then tap your big toes together. Repeat 100 times.

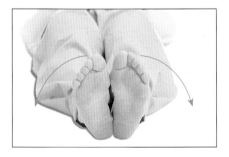

POOR EYESIGHT

Eye strain can increase stress and tension, causing the musculoskeletal system associated with eye function to become reactive. When this occurs, you might experience headaches, dizziness, gastrointestinal problems, blurry vision, redness in the eyes, photosensitivity, or pain in the eyeballs, neck, shoulders, or back.

Practitioners of Eastern Medicine correlate the eyes with the functioning of major organs, particularly the liver and kidneys. To sustain the strength of the eyes, it is important to fortify the liver and kidneys and to supply oxygen and Ki energy to the nerves that nourish the eyes.

These meridian exercises include techniques to stimulate the eyes, an important one being massage. It is extremely helpful to massage the cervical vertebrae, thereby relieving tension, fatigue, and toxic stress affecting the musculoskeletal system and your vision. These exercises help to build and sustain Ki energy flow in the liver and kidneys to augment this process.

SENDING KI ENERGY TO EYES (P. 201)

BENEFITS Reduces redness in the eyes and helps to maintain visual acuity. Relieves fatigue from the eyes and helps them to look vibrant and healthy.

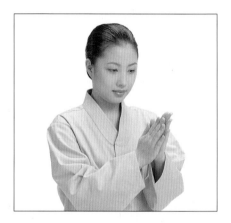

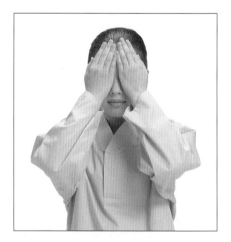

1. APPLYING PRESSURE AROUND EYES

TIPS When people experience problems with their vision, it is important to see whether, in fact, these difficulties are related to a deficiency or imbalance of Ki energy in the liver, kidneys, or heart. The meridian exercises recommended in this section are particularly beneficial in balancing the Ki energy in these organs.

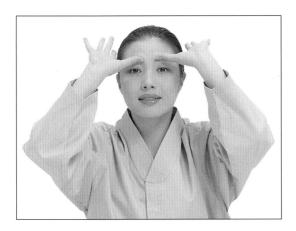

❶ With your thumbs or index fingers, gently press around the circumference of the eyes.

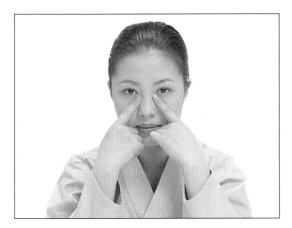

❷ With your index fingers, gently press the area under the eyes and around the bridge of the nose.

2. ROTATING EYEBALLS

BENEFITS Can help to improve vision.

Imagine looking straight ahead and viewing a triangle. Keeping your head still, rotate only your eyes to fix on the three points of the triangle. Repeat 36 times in one direction and then 36 times in the other direction.

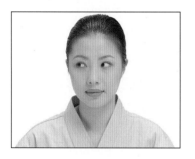
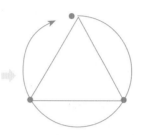

① When you first perform this exercise, begin by gazing at the bullet for one minute. Then progress to gazing at the bullet for up to 5 minutes.

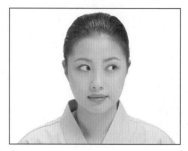
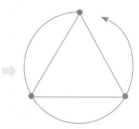

MAXIMIZE YOUR VISION

① Draw a dot on a sheet of paper and affix it to a wall. Position yourself at a 20-inch distance. Stare at the dot without blinking.

② After gazing for a while at the dot, you will notice a white halo forming around it. Keep focusing on the dot while maintaining the distinct halo.

③ You may notice redness and teardrops from your eyes in the beginning of this exercise, but keep your eyes open.

④ Now blink your eyes quickly 36 times. Then close your eyes and relax.

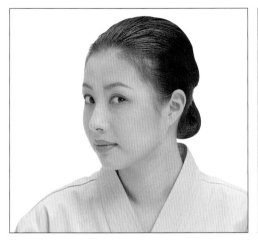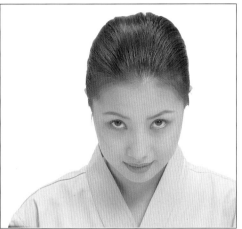

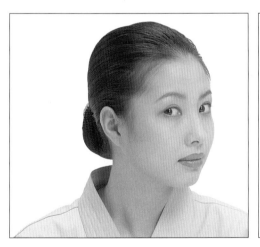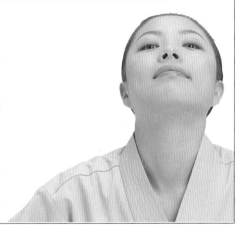

❷ Look at an imaginary dot ahead of you. Now move your head to the right while keeping your eyes straight ahead, gazing at the dot. Hold for 6 seconds and bring your head to the center for 2 seconds. Repeat to the other side.

❸ Move your head down toward your chest while holding your eyes on the bullet straight ahead of you. While still gazing at the bullet straight ahead, tilt your head backward. Keep your eyes open throughout this exercise.

IMPAIRED HEARING

Of all our sense organs, our ears move the least when we exercise, thus making health maintenance difficult. As we age, ear problems can begin to occur and hearing can progressively decline. Later on, tinnitus, or the sensation of ringing in the ears, can occur. Impaired hearing can result from a variety of causes, including cardiovascular problems, earwax, endocrinological problems, or exposure to high-pitched sounds over prolonged periods of time.

The ear has about two hundred acupressure points corresponding with our body functioning, primarily with the kidneys. Therefore, when you experience problems with your ears, it is important to strengthen the Ki energy in the kidneys, as the meridian exercises in this section instruct.

1. STIMULATING ACUPRESSURE POINTS

BENEFITS Dissipates stagnant energy around the ears, thereby strengthening the nerves. Can improve hearing and help to reduce ringing in the ears.

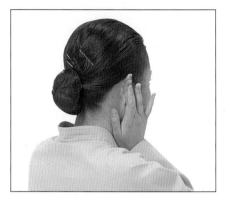

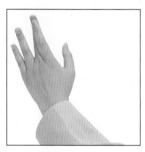

❶ Place your index finger on top of your middle finger. Place the pad of your middle finger on the cartilage of the back of your ear and fold it forward to cover the opening of your ear. With a snapping motion, move the index finger off the middle finger and tap the bone behind your ear with the index finger.

❷ Repeat this swift motion once for each year of your age. When you perform this motion rhythmically, you will hear the sound of a drum.

2. EAR PRESSING AND RELEASING WITH PALMS

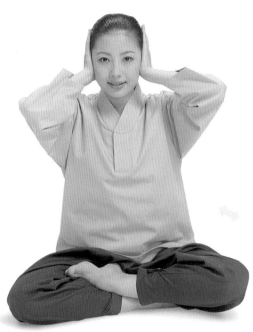

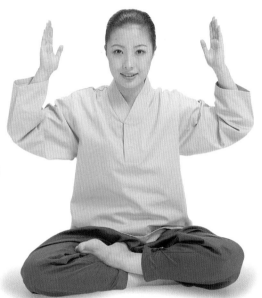

① Cover your ears with your palms. Relax your mouth and keep it slightly ajar. Apply gentle pressure. Slowly count to 3 and release quickly.

② Repeat 5 times and massage your ears. Then, with your thumbs and index fingers, gently pull on your ears in all directions to stimulate the acupressure points.

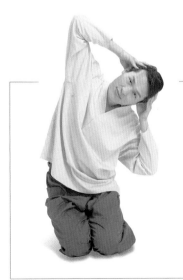

NECK ACUPRESSURE (P. 32)

INSOMNIA

Insomnia arises from an imbalance of Ki energy and blood circulation throughout the body. The Ki and blood accumulate in the head and press on the brain. Vulnerability to insomnia is commonly the result of continual stress, excessive worry, trauma, or shock. Insomnia can compromise the body's immune system and invite further ailments.

According to adherents of Eastern Medicine, the principle of Water Up, Fire Down is the requisite condition for a healthy body, mind, and spirit. When the body is not adequately rested or is undergoing intense stress, Water Up, Fire Down is thwarted and the reverse occurs: fire energy goes up toward the head, and water energy travels down toward the lower abdomen. Some of the symptoms that may occur with this are redness in the face, shoulder pain, and pain in the middle of the chest along the Conception Vessel (Im-maek), signaling a blockage of Ki energy in this area.

The recommended meridian exercises in this section emphasize relaxation and optimize the Water Up, Fire Down flow, which is crucial in alleviating insomnia.

WHOLE BODY PATTING (P. 20)

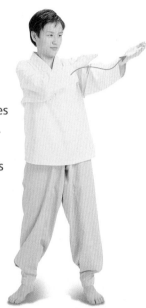

BENEFITS
Enhances blood and Ki energy circulation throughout the body and releases stagnant energy. Strengthens the cells and nervous system, helping to alleviate the problem of insomnia.

SOLE CLAPPING (P. 161)

BENEFITS Stimulates the feet and legs and helps to augment the flow of fire energy down to the lower abdomen.

TIP Relax your knee joints as you clap your feet.

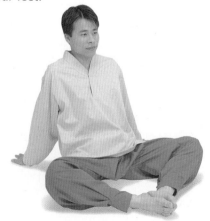

1. ENERGY MEDITATION

BENEFITS Helps to bring fire energy toward the lower abdomen for further relaxation of the body and mind.

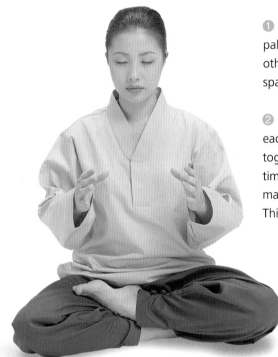

① Sit in a half-lotus position. Bring your palms in front of your chest, facing each other about 3 inches apart. Focus on the space between the hands.

② Move your hands very slowly toward each other, without touching them together, and then apart. Repeat several times. You may experience warmness or a magnetic sensation between your hands. This is Ki energy.

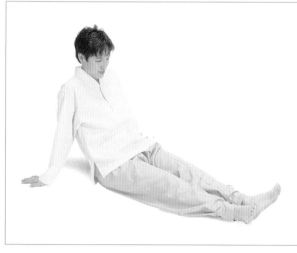

TOE TAPPING
(P. 32)

BENEFITS Releases blocked energy in the head by assisting the spontaneous flow of blood and Ki energy down to the lower abdomen to induce more restful sleep.

2. WHOLE BODY RELAXATION

BENEFITS Alleviates symptoms of heart disease, hypertension, insomnia, and headache.

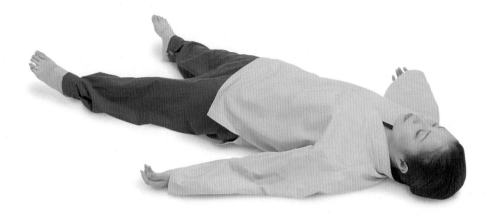

❶ Lie comfortably on your back, feet shoulder width apart and arms 45 degrees from the body. Close your eyes.

❷ Inhale slowly, deeply, and comfortably. Exhale slowly and release tension from the body. Repeat 3 times.

❸ As your eyes remain closed, begin to imagine in your mind's eye that you are observing yourself with a clear focus. You see all the parts of your body from the top of your head down to the tips of your toes.

❹ Continue to imagine that your head is becoming more and more clear and cool.

❺ Relax your facial muscles and begin to form a gentle smile. With your mind's eye, observe your smiling face.

❻ Relax your neck and shoulders completely. Imagine that stagnant energy is moving from your neck and shoulders out through your fingertips.

❼ Focus on your chest. Feel your chest expand with your breathing. Imagine your chest feeling cool and comfortable.

❽ With your mind's eye, observe your waist and abdominal area, thighs, knees, legs, ankles, and toes. As you continue to focus on your breathing, feel the calm, relaxed sensation throughout your body.

❾ As you become increasingly relaxed, imagine your body becoming heavier and heavier with each breath.

❿ Continue to breathe normally. Now, as you exhale, feel your body begin to sink deeper into the earth as you become more and more relaxed.

⓫ Imagine a very special place of peace, tranquility, and comfort just for you, provided by the whole universe.

3. STANDING THIGH STRETCH AND BALANCING

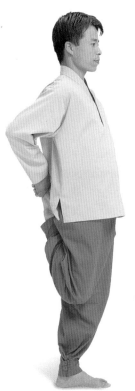

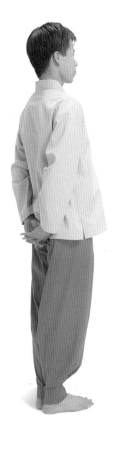

❶ Stand with your feet together. Lift your right leg behind you and grasp the top of your foot with both hands.

❷ Gently pull the top of the foot toward your hip. Relax. Repeat 10 times.

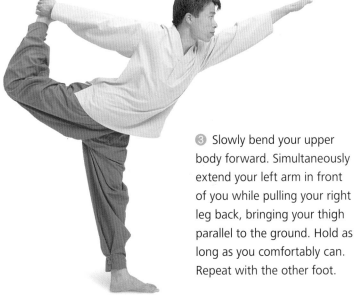

❸ Slowly bend your upper body forward. Simultaneously extend your left arm in front of you while pulling your right leg back, bringing your thigh parallel to the ground. Hold as long as you comfortably can. Repeat with the other foot.

4. OPENING THE CHEST

BENEFITS Helps to release stagnant fire energy from the chest. It is beneficial for insomnia and headache.

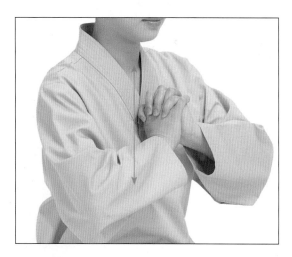

❶ Sit in a half-lotus position, or stand. Interlace your fingers at chest level and tap your chest with your thumb knuckles, moving up and down from the chest to the throat area.

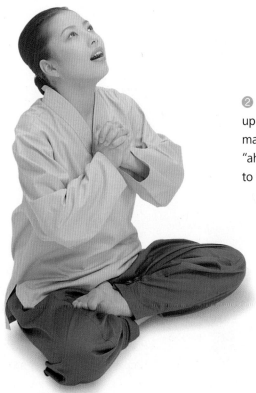

❷ Lift up your chin. Open up your mouth and begin to make the continuous sound of "ahhhhhhhh" as you continue to tap up and down.

5. BRIDGE POSTURE VARIATION

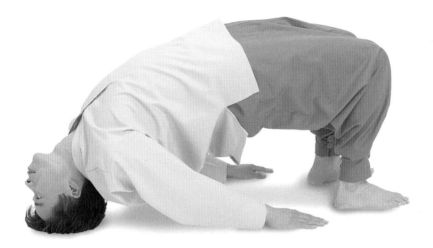

❶ Lie on your back, bend your knees so your feet are flat on the floor, and inhale. Let your hands rest on the floor near your sides. Lift your hips and raise your chin, placing your body weight on the top of your head. Hold for as long as you comfortably can.

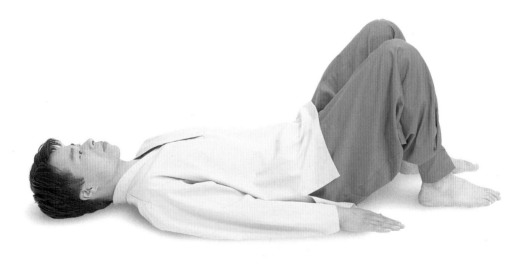

❷ Continue to hold this posture until you begin to feel your face flush. Quickly drop your hips down to the floor, while at the same time making the sound "hoht." Repeat 3 times.

6. BUTTOCK TAPPING

BENEFITS Assists in circulating blood from the lower extremities to the head. Cools the head and calms the mind.

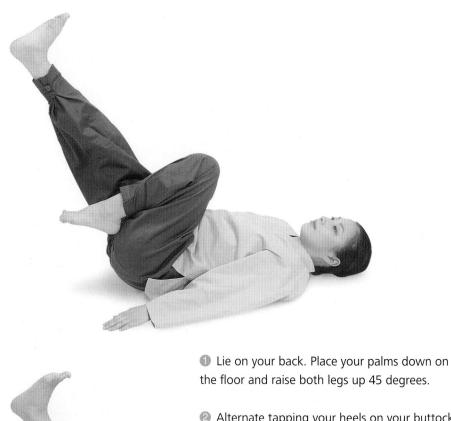

❶ Lie on your back. Place your palms down on the floor and raise both legs up 45 degrees.

❷ Alternate tapping your heels on your buttocks 30 times.

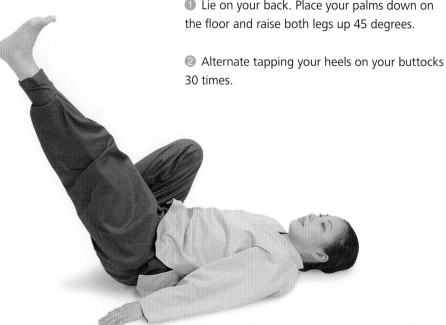

7. SEATED ANKLE ROTATION

BENEFITS Relaxes waist and legs. Enables blood and Ki energy to circulate throughout the body.

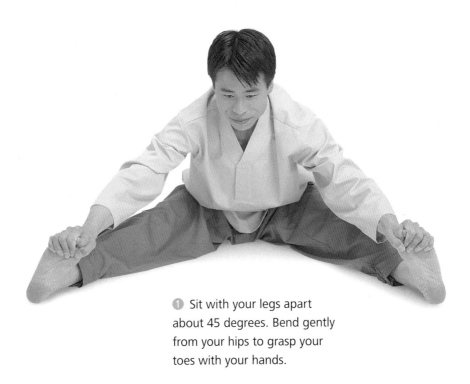

❶ Sit with your legs apart about 45 degrees. Bend gently from your hips to grasp your toes with your hands.

❷ Rotate toes in a circular manner, first inward and then outward.

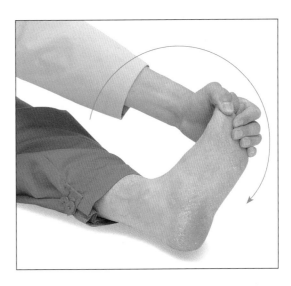

HANGOVER

Alcohol consumption is often accompanied by breath odor and a headache. Eventually the alcohol evaporates and the smell dissipates. It is important to release the toxins caused by alcohol from the body as quickly as possible.

Abdominal breathing is not advised after generous consumption of alcohol. In its effort to filter the toxins from the body, the liver, already weakened by stress and fatigue, is further taxed as it attempts to detoxify the effects of the alcohol. Abdominal breathing alone could cause an increase in the circulation of the alcohol throughout the body, causing more effort for the liver to detoxify the body. Instead, it is recommended to perform deep breathing along with the meridian exercises in this section. This will open the liver meridian channels to enhance energy circulation in the liver, thus assisting in the process of detoxification from the effects of the alcohol.

WHOLE BODY PATTING (P. 20)

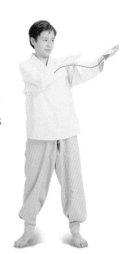

BENEFITS Enhances circulation of Ki and blood throughout the body and releases stagnant toxins. Helps to eliminate insomnia and strengthens the nervous system and the cells throughout the body.

SOLE CLAPPING (P. 161)

BENEFITS Stimulates the feet and legs as it brings fire energy toward the lower abdomen.

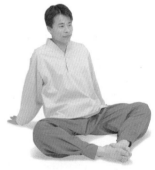

SEATED SIDE BEND (P. 197)

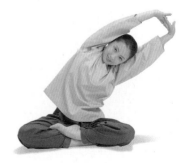

1. DEEP BREATHING

BENEFITS Enables quick alcohol evaporation from the bloodstream.

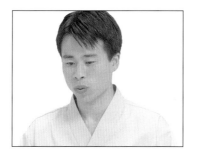

❶ Inhale slowly and deeply through your nose to the lower abdomen. Exhale slowly and completely through your mouth. Repeat this 10 times.

2. OPENING MERIDIANS IN THE LEGS

BENEFITS Opens the Liver and Gall Bladder Meridians and enhances liver and gall bladder functioning. Helps to quickly detoxify the alcohol from the body.

❶ Sit on the floor. Bend your knees and relax your legs. Using either your palms or your fists, pat your leg from the top of your thigh down to the ankle. Use one hand on the outside of your leg and the other on the inside, and continue to pat up and down. Repeat 2-3 times.

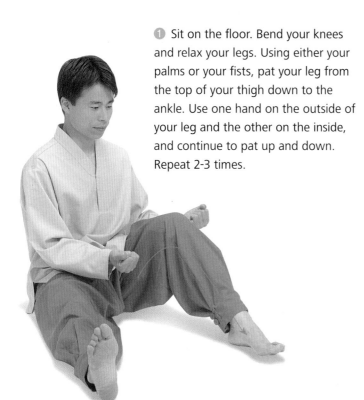

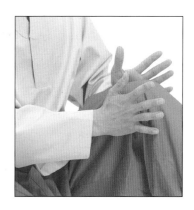

❷ Place your palms on either side of one knee and gently massage with a circular motion. Follow this by sweeping downward. Repeat with the other leg.

3. CHEST OPENING

TIP Keep your elbows at a 90-degree angle.

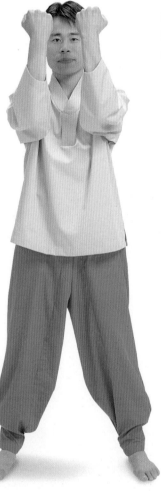

❶ Stand with your feet shoulder width apart. Bring your elbows in front of your face at 90-degree angles.

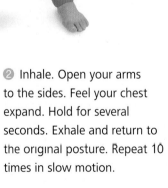

❷ Inhale. Open your arms to the sides. Feel your chest expand. Hold for several seconds. Exhale and return to the original posture. Repeat 10 times in slow motion.

4. SIDE LEG LIFT FOR LIVER

BENEFITS Enhances the Liver and Gall Bladder Meridian functioning to enable rapid evaporation of alcohol toxins from the body. Helps to lessen fatigue.

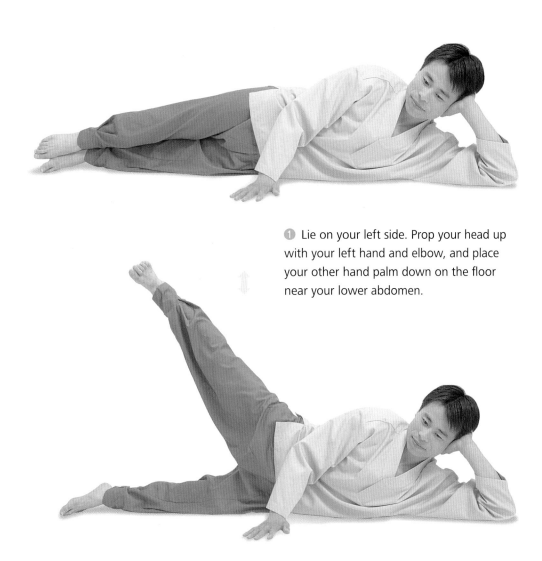

❶ Lie on your left side. Prop your head up with your left hand and elbow, and place your other hand palm down on the floor near your lower abdomen.

❷ Gently lift and lower your leg without bending your knee. Repeat 20 times. Then switch legs and repeat 20 more times.

5. CHEST ACUPRESSURE

BENEFITS Opens the chest, relieving fatigue in the liver and tightness in the chest.

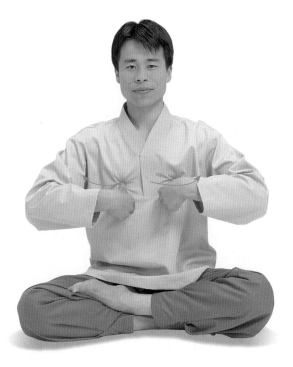

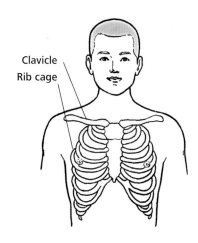

Clavicle
Rib cage

❶ Sit in a half-lotus position. Place your thumbs near the center of your chest in the space between the clavicle and the solar plexus, and press. Move your thumbs outward along the same rib and continue to press.

❷ Reposition your thumbs on the next rib below, and press again from the center in the space between the bones of the ribs and moving outward. Proceed downward toward the bottom of the rib cage.

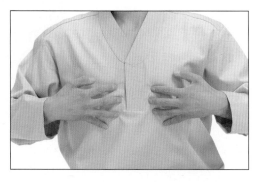

❸ Spread your fingers and place them between the bones of the top 6 ribs. Exhale and simultaneously press. Continue this motion as you move down your rib cage, making certain to cover the spaces between each of your ribs.

6. SPINE TWISTING

BENEFITS Stimulates the Tenth Thoracic Vertebra to enhance liver and kidney function. Detoxifies as it enables more rapid excretion of water from the body.

❶ Sit on the floor with your right leg bent and your foot near your left hip. Bend your left leg and place the foot flat on the floor near your right knee.

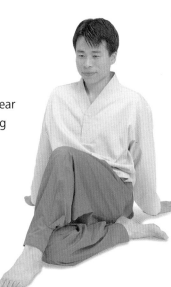

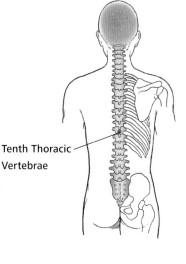

Tenth Thoracic Vertebrae

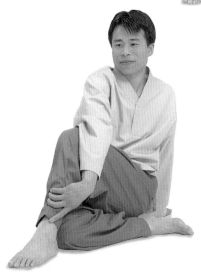

❷ Place your right arm on the outside of your left knee and grasp the outside of your left ankle.

❸ Inhale while maintaining a straight, but not rigid, spine. Turn your upper body to the left and follow the movement with your eyes. Focus on your spine. Exhale and gently return to center.

❹ Alternate sides and repeat 3 times each.

FATIGUE

Chronic fatigue can result from lack of sleep, overwork, malnutrition, or excessive stress. It can also be a symptom of liver disease or fatty deposits in the liver, impeding proper Ki circulation, which is vital for good health. If you are experiencing chronic fatigue, you may find that even if you rest, you still feel tired. Symptoms such as pain and stiffness—particularly in the neck, shoulders, and lower back—and a general heaviness in the body signal to adherents of Eastern Medicine that there are blockages in the acupressure points and meridians.

The recommended meridian exercises in this section will help to release the stagnant Ki energy that has become blocked, revitalizing energy and reducing fatigue.

LEG SWEEP
(P. 97)

BENEFITS Stimulates the Urinary Bladder Meridian, relieving fatigue in the waist and legs.

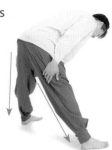

INNER THIGH STRETCH
(P. 126)

BENEFITS Enables fire energy to come down to the lower abdomen to enable more peaceful and restful sleep.

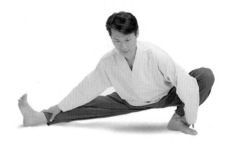

BICYCLE EXERCISE
(P. 140)

BENEFITS Strengthens lower extremities and stimulates the muscles and nerves around the perineal and reproductive glands. Enhances stamina; enables more effective blood and Ki energy circulation in the head. Relieves fatigue from the lower extremities.

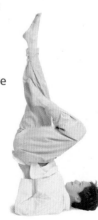

ROLLING BOW POSTURE (P. 214)

BENEFITS Stimulates the spine and the central nervous system, realigns the spine, and enhances endocrine gland function. Speeds recovery from chronic general fatigue. Beneficial for those spending prolonged hours sitting or in other sedentary positions.

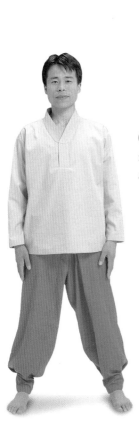

OPENING MERIDIANS IN THE LEGS (P. 305)

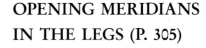

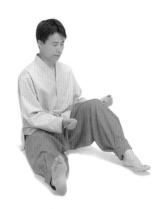

1. STRETCHING ARMS TO THE SKY

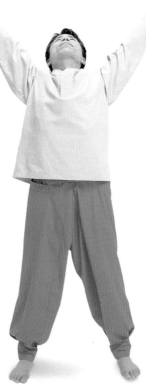

❶ Stand with your legs shoulder width and your arms at your sides.

❷ Inhale. Keeping your fingers together, expand your chest as you stretch your arms above your head toward the sky. Keep your elbows soft but not bent. Your weight should be felt on your toes.

❸ Exhale to STEP 1, and repeat once more.

2. PUSHING ENERGY WITH THE HANDS TOWARD THE SKY AND THE EARTH

BENEFITS Helps one to recover from fatigue as the strong energy from heaven and earth is received in the body.

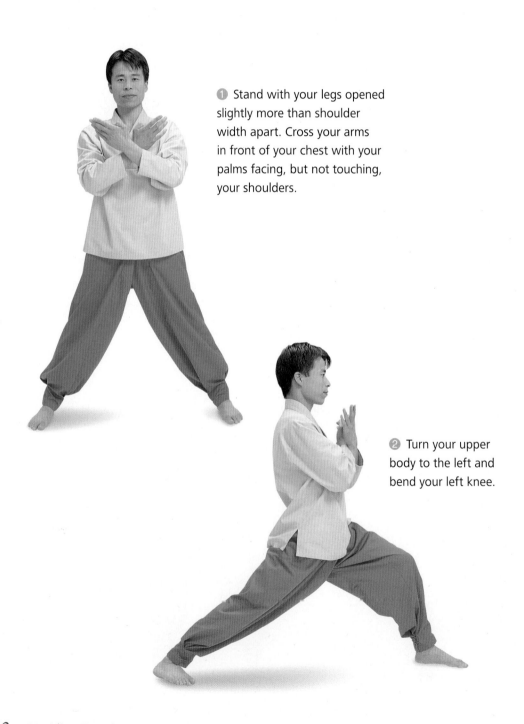

❶ Stand with your legs opened slightly more than shoulder width apart. Cross your arms in front of your chest with your palms facing, but not touching, your shoulders.

❷ Turn your upper body to the left and bend your left knee.

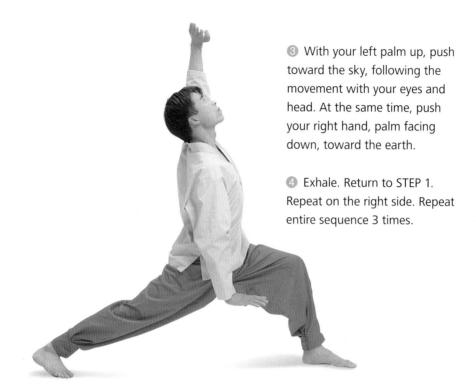

③ With your left palm up, push toward the sky, following the movement with your eyes and head. At the same time, push your right hand, palm facing down, toward the earth.

④ Exhale. Return to STEP 1. Repeat on the right side. Repeat entire sequence 3 times.

SOLE CLAPPING
(P. 161)

LEG LIFT AND TWIST
(P. 240)

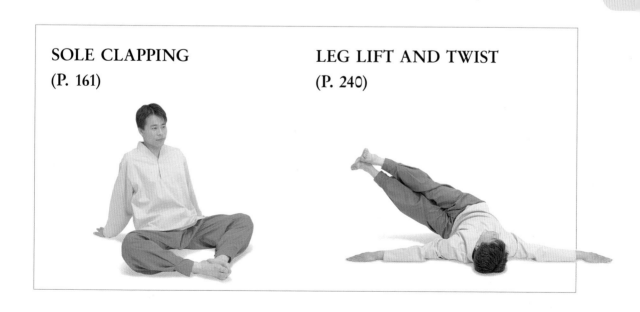

SPRING FATIGUE

People often notice that as the spring season approaches, they are not as energetic as they would like to be. Adherents of Eastern Medicine believe this is due to the fluctuation in the biorhythms of the body.

In the wintertime, muscles are contracted, and Ki energy and blood circulation are more constricted. In the change from winter to spring, the organs increase their functioning capacity and need more energy. People who do not participate in appropriate exercise during the winter have less Ki energy accumulated for spring. They find adjusting to the change of seasons arduous and can experience significant spring fatigue.

The most significant symptoms signaling spring fatigue are lethargy, decrease in appetite, digestive problems, and dizziness. The meridian exercises in this section are designed to increase vitality.

TIPTOE STRETCH
(P. 236)

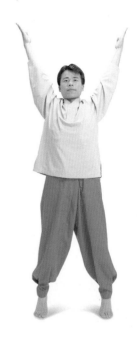

REACH, TWIST, AND BEND
(P. 122)

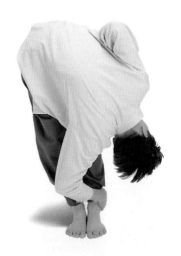

1. PUSHING KI ENERGY

BENEFITS Assists in sending Ki energy from the lower abdomen throughout the body. Also helps to release toxins from the body.

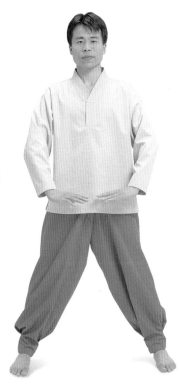

① Stand with your feet more than shoulder width apart and bend your knees over your toes. Inhale and slowly bring your hands, palms up, toward your chest.

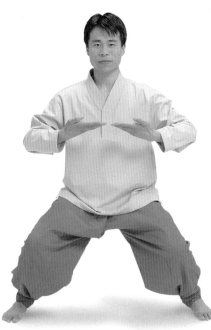

② Hold your breath as you slowly push your palms out to the sides.

③ Hold and then bring your hands to your lower abdomen, palms down. Exhale and bring your hands down to your sides.

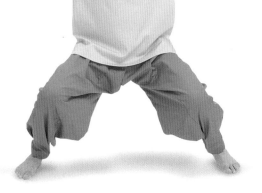

2. CIRCLE STRETCH

BENEFITS Enhances organ function. Helps to release stagnant blood from the abdomen and to facilitate Ki energy flow.

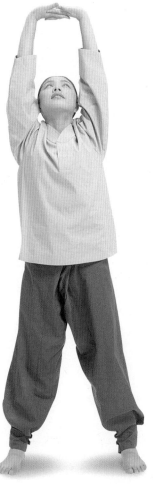

❶ Stand with your feet shoulder width apart. Inhale and interlace your fingers. Raise them above your head with your palms facing the sky and follow the movement with your eyes. Hold your breath.

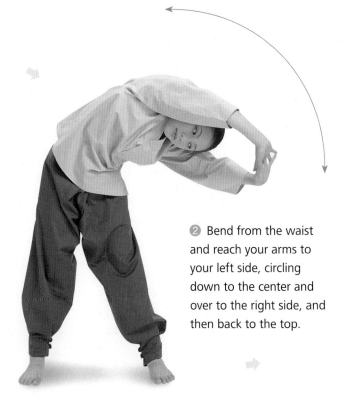

❷ Bend from the waist and reach your arms to your left side, circling down to the center and over to the right side, and then back to the top.

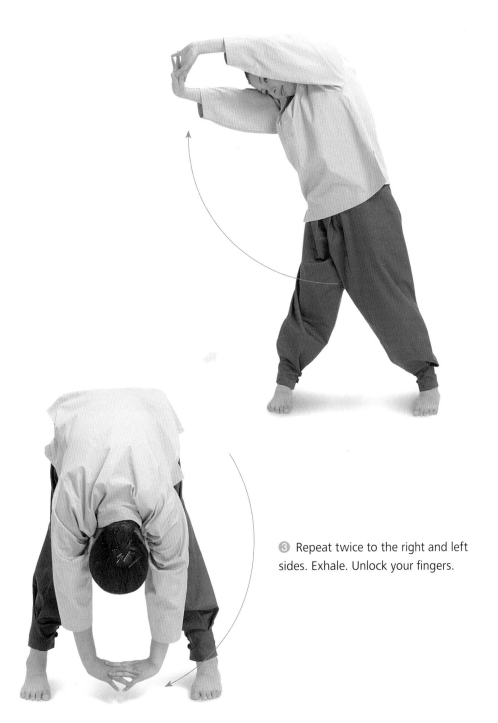

❸ Repeat twice to the right and left sides. Exhale. Unlock your fingers.

Other Conditions   *317*

3. SITTING HAMSTRING STRETCH

TIPS Keep your knee straight but soft and tilt your head back.

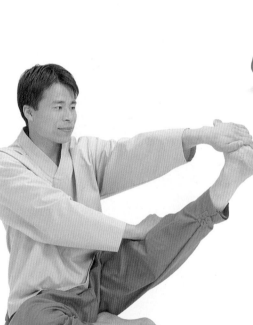

❶ Sit on the floor or on a chair. With your left hand, grasp the bottom of your left foot.

❷ Keeping hold of your foot, extend your left leg at shoulder height. Place your right hand on your left knee with slight pressure as you stretch.

❸ Gently tilt your head backward, following with your eyes. Hold for several seconds and release.

❹ Repeat this exercise with your right leg. Perform 2 more times with each leg.

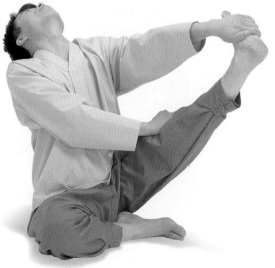

SPRING FATIGUE

4. FORWARD BEND WITH CLASPED HANDS

TIPS Keep your knees straight but soft. When you bend your upper body, straighten your arms and bring them forward without locking them.

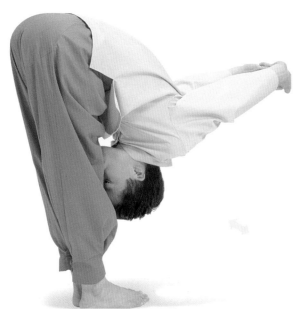

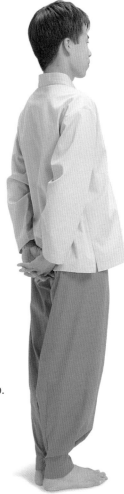

❶ Stand with your feet together and interlace your fingers behind you. Inhale. Bend your torso forward, bringing your head toward your knees. Drop your shoulders, letting your arms swing out behind you, and relax.

❷ Exhale. Slowly stand up. Repeat 3 times.

appendix

1. The Spine, Main Pillar of Our Body

2. Position of Organs and the Skeleton

3. Meridians, Rivers of Ki Energy

1. THE SPINE, MAIN PILLAR OF OUR BODY

The spinal column, pillar of the human body, consists of seven cervical vertebrae, twelve thoracic vertebrae, five lumbar vertebrae, the sacrum (five fused vertebrae), and the coccyx (four fused vertebrae) in descending order. The entire spinal column, which consists of thirty-three vertebrae, is S-shaped.

Since autonomic nerves corresponding to each organ travel throughout the spinal column, problems in the spine have an impact on the organs as well. When the cervical vertebrae are injured, the disks put pressure on the nerves, which can cause pain anywhere in the body. Nerves that branch out of the thoracic vertebrae connect to the five viscera (solid organs) and six entrails (hollow organs) and regulate functions of the internal organs.

Poor posture and bad habits threaten the health of the lower back and spine. For example, sitting with the hip pulled forward, sitting with legs crossed, and talking on the phone with your head bent to one side are all detrimental to your spine. It is important to form habits such as sitting with the spine straight and making sure that you bend your knees when you lift a heavy item.

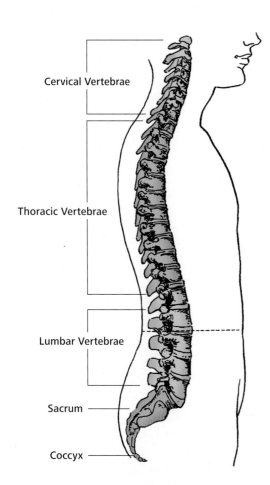

Cervical Vertebrae

Thoracic Vertebrae

Lumbar Vertebrae

Sacrum

Coccyx

When you do meridian exercises regularly, it is possible to correct a misaligned spinal column with pulling and stretching movements. The healthy spine is reflected in the overall well-being of the body.

Violent movement, sudden shock, or poor posture can damage the disks in the spinal column. When this occurs, the damaged disk may exert pressure on the nerves, causing extreme pain throughout the body and inhibiting movement of the spine itself.

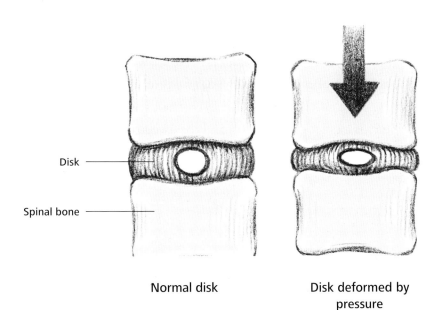

Disk

Spinal bone

Normal disk

Disk deformed by pressure

2. POSITION OF ORGANS AND THE SKELETON

Can you accurately point to where the stomach is located in the body? Is the liver located on the right or the left side? Understanding the body's structure and functions, including positions of the organs and skeleton, is helpful when doing meridian exercises.

When you send energy to a specific organ or problem area, the more accurately you can imagine the position or the shape of the organ, the greater the effect will be. It's also important to understand the specific function of each organ. The liver is the chemical factory of our body, the stomach is a factory where food is broken down and processed, and the heart is a pump that circulates blood throughout the whole body. When you do meridian exercises, you should wholeheartedly thank these hard-working organs.

Bones support the body and protect the internal organs. The skull protects the brain, and the ribs encircle the heart and lungs. Bone marrow is located inside the bones and generates red blood cells that deliver oxygen and nutrients to the body and white blood cells that destroy harmful bacteria. When your body moves, focus on each movement. Begin observing your body and you will find that you are also observing your mind. In other words, we can reach the mind through the body. The body is a mirror of the mind and the dwelling place of the soul.

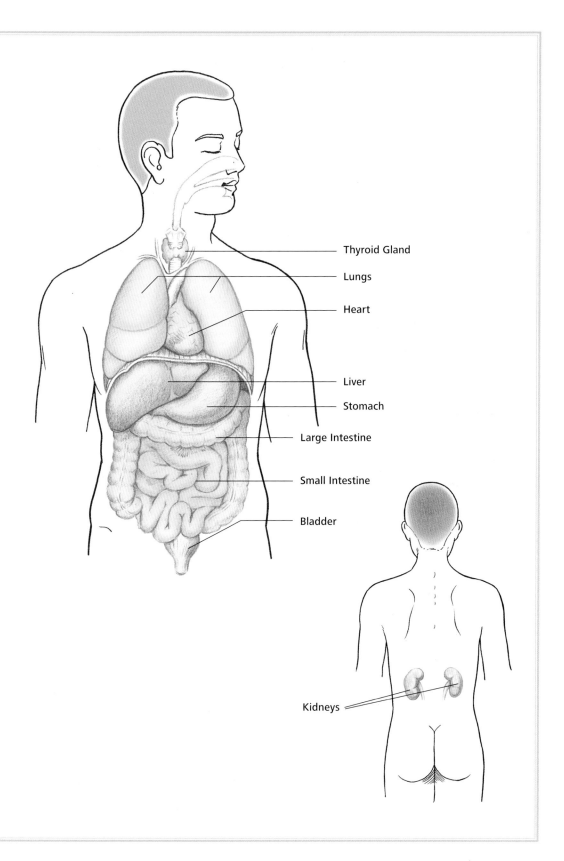

Thyroid Gland

Lungs

Heart

Liver

Stomach

Large Intestine

Small Intestine

Bladder

Kidneys

3. MERIDIANS, RIVERS OF KI ENERGY

Meridians and acupressure points are an invisible network of life energy, pathways through which Ki energy travels the body. There are twelve main meridians and 365 primary acupressure points in the human body.

The twelve main meridians are Lung, Large Intestine, Stomach, Spleen, Heart, Small Intestine, Bladder, Kidney, Pericardium, Triple Burner, Gall Bladder, and Liver. They travel bilaterally in the right and left sides of the body, connecting the organs. Even the sole of the foot is connected to every organ of the body.

In the perspective of Eastern Medicine, disease is created because the flow of Ki energy that travels through meridians and acupressure points is blocked and imbalanced, so the goal of meridian exercise is to open the passageways so Ki energy can flow freely.

As few as nine or as many as sixty acupressure points are distributed along a single meridian, but you don't have to memorize all of them. Simply grasping a basic understanding of the general flow of a meridian can help you to achieve the goal of meridian exercise. For example, when you have problems in the liver, simply tapping, massaging, applying pressure, or stroking along the liver meridian will be highly effective. If you practice long enough, you will sense electricity along the meridians, proving you've mastered meridian exercise.

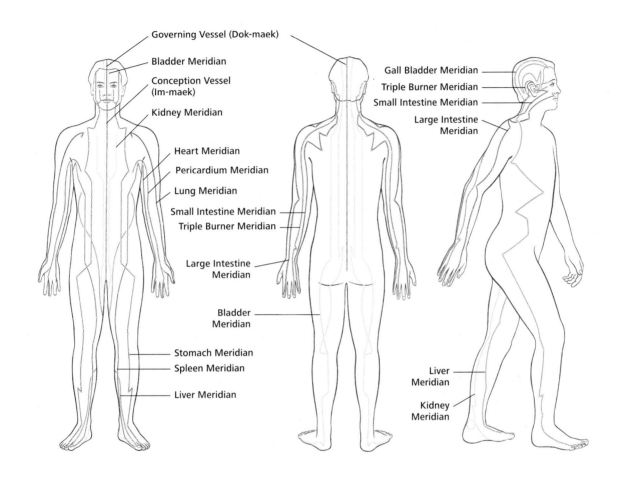

Governing Vessel (Dok-maek)

Bladder Meridian

Conception Vessel (Im-maek)

Kidney Meridian

Heart Meridian

Pericardium Meridian

Lung Meridian

Small Intestine Meridian

Triple Burner Meridian

Large Intestine Meridian

Bladder Meridian

Stomach Meridian

Spleen Meridian

Liver Meridian

Gall Bladder Meridian

Triple Burner Meridian

Small Intestine Meridian

Large Intestine Meridian

Liver Meridian

Kidney Meridian

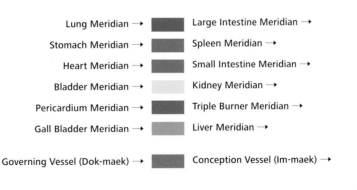

Lung Meridian →

Stomach Meridian →

Heart Meridian →

Bladder Meridian →

Pericardium Meridian →

Gall Bladder Meridian →

Governing Vessel (Dok-maek) →

Large Intestine Meridian →

Spleen Meridian →

Small Intestine Meridian →

Kidney Meridian →

Triple Burner Meridian →

Liver Meridian →

Conception Vessel (Im-maek) →

1) LUNG MERIDIAN

SYMPTOMS OF BLOCKED ENERGY: difficulty breathing, asthma, tightness in the chest

When the lungs, which assimilate air and distribute oxygen to the five main organs, weaken, the flow of the Lung Meridian is easily blocked. When there are problems in the Lung Meridian, the function of all respiratory organs (nose, throat, lungs, and bronchi) are impaired as well. You may experience a hot face, dry mouth, stifling feeling in the chest, aching arms and legs, or sweaty palms. As the function of the lungs deteriorates, you may appear listless or your skin may be dull. Under these conditions, applying pressure to the acupressure points along the Lung Meridian facilitates the flow of energy and revitalizes the organs.

2) LARGE INTESTINE MERIDIAN

SYMPTOMS OF BLOCKED ENERGY: yellowish eyes, sore throat, stuffy nose, toothache, pain along the shoulders and arms

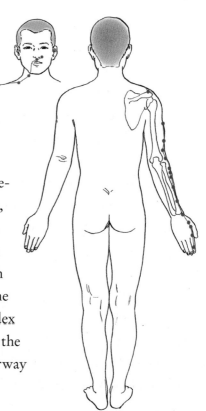

Symptoms of problems with the Large Intestine Meridian are found in the face, shoulders, or arms, with pain often concentrated in the index fingers. In this case, give a finger pressure treatment along the flow of the Large Intestine Meridian. Start with your index finger pointed upward and press on the meridian at your wrist, in line with the pointed index finger. Continue to press along the meridian up to the clavicle and lightly press on the area next to the airway on both sides.

3) STOMACH MERIDIAN

SYMPTOMS OF BLOCKED ENERGY: sores around the mouth, tension in the jaws, headache in the area of the eyes or sinuses, pain in the abdominal area or on the sides of the lower limbs

Problems in the Stomach Meridian result in headaches with severe pain, particularly in the forehead, around the eyes, or in the back of the head. Other symptoms include stuffy nose and occasional nosebleeds. Skin tone may become lusterless and dull. Lips may be dry or articulation poor. In this case, tapping the St 36 (Jok-sam-lee) points or toe tapping is beneficial. Also, relax and lightly tap along the Stomach Meridian from the side of the head to the front of the ear to the cheek in a straight line.

4) SPLEEN MERIDIAN

SYMPTOMS OF BLOCKED ENERGY: nausea, frequent belching

The spleen is mainly responsible for digestion. When the spleen functions well, digestion is good and there is abundant Ki energy and blood in the body. However, when the spleen is out of balance, you may experience lack of energy or insufficient blood in some or all parts of your body. You may have poor digestion, causing stomachaches, diarrhea, or a loss of appetite.

When the spleen is lethargic, your tongue may stiffen or you may feel pain and heaviness above the stomach. You may also feel intestinal upset, indigestion, frequent constipation, cold legs, or stiffness in the knees. Women may experience abnormal periods, occasional irregular uterine bleeding or insomnia. For these symptoms, it is beneficial to stimulate the Ki 1 (Yong-chun) acupressure points daily and to press along the Spleen Meridian with your thumb.

5) HEART MERIDIAN

SYMPTOMS OF BLOCKED ENERGY: pain below the solar plexus, in the upper chest, or in the upper part of the arm

The Heart Meridian governs functioning of the heart and regulates brain function. Bloodshot eyes, a dry throat, and insomnia are indications of problems with the heart. The area below the solar plexus may be painful, and there may be acute pain in the arms and little fingers. A flushed face is also a common symptom of problems along the Heart Meridian. You could experience strong pulsing in the side of the head, neck, wrists, top of the foot, or stomach. Uncontrollable emotions and fatigue are common as well. Under these conditions, if you press below the solar plexus and inside the shoulder blades, you will feel pain and may find swelling or lumps. For these symptoms, tap the depression between the breasts with your fingertips or fist and then tap the Heart Meridian from the armpit down the arm to the little finger.

6) SMALL INTESTINE MERIDIAN

SYMPTOMS OF BLOCKED ENERGY: hearing difficulty, urinary disorders, yellowish eyes

The Small Intestine Meridian regulates the small intestine, which is in charge of the absorption of nutrients. The small intestine acts as a filter between pure and stale energy, receiving food from the stomach and absorbing energy from the food after the digestive processes. During this process, pure energy transfers to the spleen and stale energy to the large intestine. When you have problems with the small intestine, the whites of the eyes become yellow and hearing becomes less acute. The head can feel heavy and the arms ache or feel chilled. For these symptoms, extend your arm with your palm down and apply finger pressure on the Small Intestine Meridian between the wrist and the base of the little finger, proceeding on up the back of the arm.

7) BLADDER MERIDIAN

SYMPTOMS OF BLOCKED ENERGY: pain and tension in eyes and neck, fever and chills, nasal congestion, eye disease, lower back pain, cramps in the backs of the legs, urinary difficulties

Problems with the Bladder Meridian are reflected in pain in the eyes, neck, back, or the backs of the legs. This meridian also affects reproductive functioning. Acupressure points along the sides of the spine are extremely important and quickly signal problems arising in the internal organs. For menopausal symptoms or problems in the reproductive organs, regulate the Bladder Meridian. Stretch the legs forward and alternately shake each leg. You can also bend your upper body forward to activate the Bladder Meridian.

8) KIDNEY MERIDIAN

SYMPTOMS OF BLOCKED ENERGY: dark and rough complexion, dry mouth, swollen throat, shortness of breath

The first sign of weakening of the Kidney Meridian is pain or weakness in the back or knees. The kidney regulates reproductive function and urination, so problems may appear as diarrhea, sexual dysfunction, loss of appetite, or general weakness. A simple but effective way to activate the Kidney Meridian is to hit or apply pressure to the Ki 1 (Yong-chun) points, located on the soles of the feet, with your fist or thumb. With the lower back straight and both hands on your lower abdomen, inhale deeply as you gently push your stomach out. As you exhale, pull your stomach in as if to touch the spine.

9) PERICARDIUM MERIDIAN

SYMPTOMS OF BLOCKED ENERGY: mental restlessness, palpitations, a flushed face, tightness in the chest, heat sensation in the palms

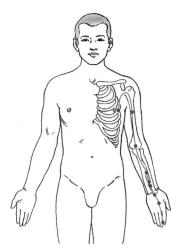

The pericardium is a mass of energy that wraps the heart like a scarf and is often called the heart protector. The Pericardium Meridian has many symptoms in common with the Heart Meridian. Lightly tap the Pericardium Meridian, which flows from the chest, through the middle of the inside of the arms, to the inside of the middle finger.

10) TRIPLE BURNER MERIDIAN

SYMPTOMS OF BLOCKED ENERGY: pain along the lines of ear, eye, face, jaw, neck, shoulder, arm, top of the hand, and fourth finger

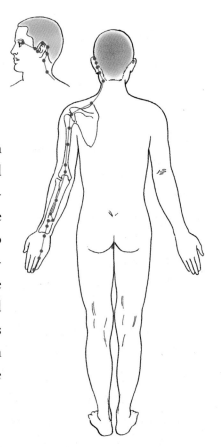

The Triple Burner Meridian is associated with the membrane that covers the internal organs and protects them. The upper burner runs from below the neck to below the diaphragm, the middle burner includes the area from the diaphragm to the navel, and the lower burner runs from the navel to the groin area. All three together constitute the Triple Burner Meridian. A breathing method that revives the meridian, a source of the body's energy supply, is abdominal breathing. Place both hands on your lower abdomen and breathe while focusing on your Dahn-jon.

11) GALL BLADDER MERIDIAN

SYMPTOMS OF BLOCKED ENERGY: temporal headaches; migraines; or problems in the face, ears, skin, armpits, knees, or the outer legs or feet

The Gall Bladder Meridian encircles a large area—from the head to the feet on both sides of the body. When you suffer from headaches or have problems in the face, skin, or legs, taking good care of the Gall Bladder Meridian is very effective. Problems in the liver or the gall bladder can cause a bluish look in the whites of the eye, low energy with a feeble voice, or a high-pitched voice. For these symptoms, practice meridian exercises that stimulate the Gall Bladder Meridian, which flows through the sides of the body from the outer eye to the ear, from the temple area over the top of the head to the top of the shoulder, and from the side down to the buttocks, down the outer thigh, and down the leg to the fourth toe.

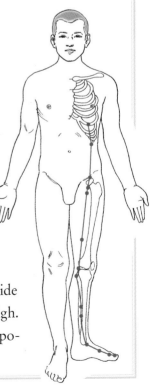

12) LIVER MERIDIAN

SYMPTOMS OF BLOCKED ENERGY: dull complexion, dry throat, nausea, a feeling of heaviness in the chest, anger, painful red eyes and face

Problems with liver function can have wide-ranging effects, both physically and emotionally. Because the Liver Meridian connects directly to the reproductive organs in both men and women, treating it is effective for problems related to the reproductive organs. The Liver Meridian flows from the big toe, up the foot, and through the middle of the inside of each leg. With your legs stretched out, tap along the inside edge of the top of your foot and move up to the inside of the thigh. It is also effective to tap your toe tips together while in a sitting position with your hands on your lower abdomen.

Symptom/Benefit Index

A

anxiety 30–39, 164–169, 269

appetite 178–189

arthritis 120, 128–133, 146, 203

autonomic nervous system difficulties
    44–51

B

Bell's Palsy 40–43

bladder infection 230–233

blushing 84

bone marrow 52, 135, 185

bronchitis 88, 137, 189

C

cholesterol 95, 150, 174

cold 88–95

cold congestion 89

concentration 34, 38–39, 177

constipation 208–215

cough 88

D–E

diabetes 68–77, 274

diarrhea 204–207, 329

emphysema 89

F

facial nerve disorders 40–43

fatigue 310–313

flu 88–95

focus 34, 39, 68, 151, 167

G

gastrointestinal disorders 178–189

H

hair loss 146–149

hangovers 304–309

headaches 30–39, 269

heart disorders 150–163

hemorrhoids 218 – 221

hot flashes 84

hypertension (high blood pressure)
    164–169

hypotension (low blood pressure)
    170–173

I

impaired hearing 294–195

insomnia 269, 296–303

itchiness 27, 142

K

knee pain 273

kidney disorders 222–229

L

lethargy 310–313

leucorrhea 264–271

liver disorders 190–203

lower back pain 96–107

lumbago 97, 107, 230, 240, 275

lung disorders 78–87

M

menstrual cramps 272–273

menstrual disorders 272–277

N

neck pain 108–111

numbness 52–55

O

obesity 278–289

osteoporosis 134–135

P

pneumonia 137, 189

poor eyesight 290–293

post partum 260–263

pregnancy 242–259

R

reproductive system 68, 211, 237,
    240, 260, 282

S

sciatic pain 120–127

sciatica 120, 182

sexual dysfunction 230, 234, 237, 265

shoulder pain 42, 108, 112–119

skin disorders 136–145

skin radiance 272

spasms 120, 134, 183, 272

spring fatigue 314–319

stamina 234–241, 269

stroke 174–177

T

thyroid disorders 56–57

U

ulcers 182

uterine bleeding 273, 329

Products of Related Interest

Home Healing Massage: Hwal-gong for Everyday Wellness
Institute of Human Technology

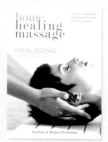

A comprehensive guide to the natural healing power of touch based on ancient Korean massage techniques, this book will give you increased ability to develop total wellness for yourself and your family. Each fully-illustrated chapter provides a complete overview of energy principles and massage techniques that effectively alleviate many common ailments. Most of all, you will be able to experience the sheer joy of giving and receiving love through the act of hands-on healing.

Body & Brain Yoga Essentials: Featuring Brain Wave Vibration
Instructed by Dawn Quaresima

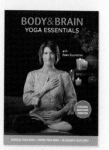

Develop a strong and flexible body, boost your energy and vitality, and bring balance back into your life with the basic Body & Brain Yoga class on this DVD. Let certified, nationally-famous instructor Dawn Quaresima guide you through a one-hour training session that includes meridian exercises, meditative breathing techniques, and an energy awareness meditation.

Magnetic Meditation Kit: 5 Minutes to Health, Energy and Clarity
Ilchi Lee

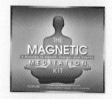

Magnetic Meditation is a groundbreaking method of meditation in which you use the tangible sensation of the magnetic fields of magnets to feel, amplify, and circulate energy. Meditating for just 5 minutes with magnets will totally change your meditation experiences. This kit includes an illustrated instructional book and three magnets.

The Power Brain: Five Steps to Upgrading Your Brain Operating System   *Ilchi Lee*

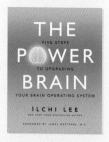

Author Ilchi Lee teaches readers how to take control of their brains in five simple steps, thus making it easier for them to achieve their dreams. This book is the most comprehensive presentation of his world-renown Brain Education method, which uses simple mind-body techniques, such as meridian exercise, emotional renewal exercises, and energy meditations, to release the brain's creative and cognitive potential.

Find these and all Best Life Media products at BestLifeMedia.com.